THE ALKALINE DIET

FOR MEN Cookbook

The Best **120+** Recipes to Stay
HEALTHY and **FIT** with Alkaline Diet!

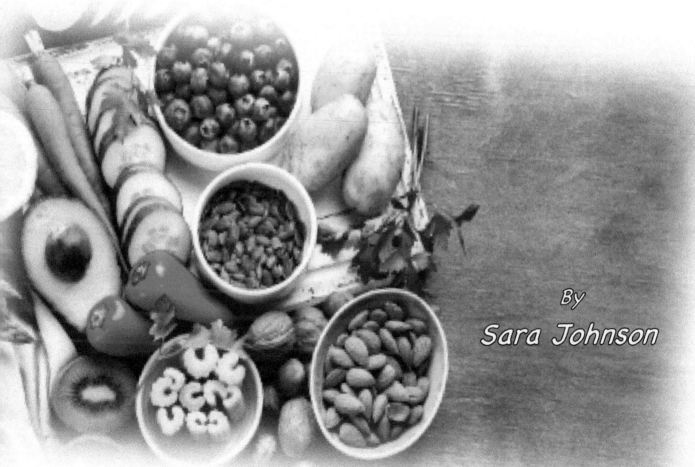

By

Sara Johnson

Table of Contents

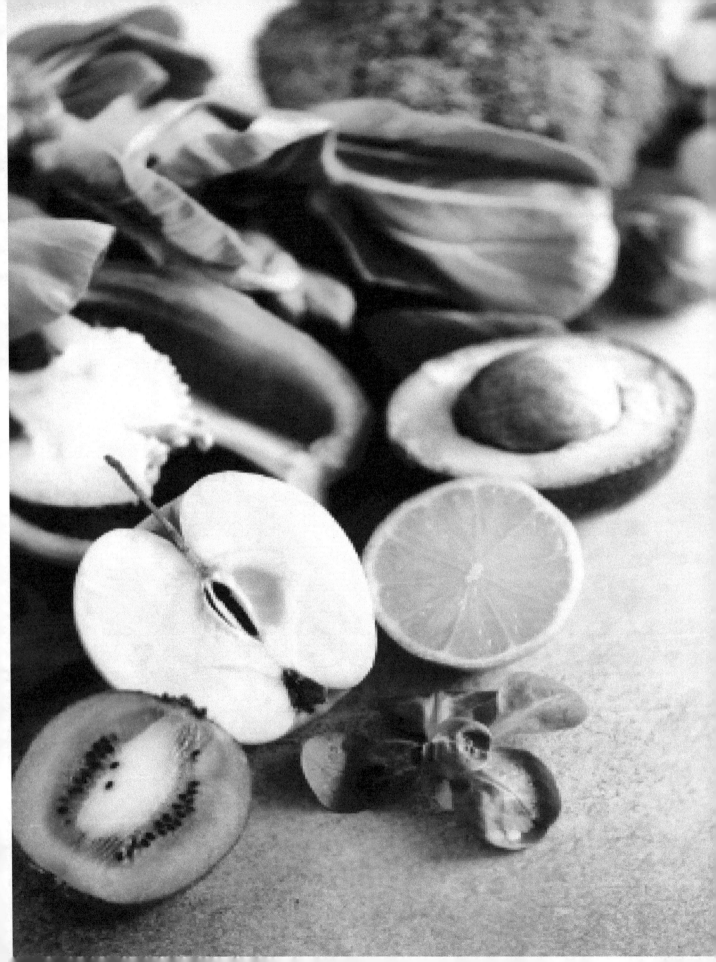

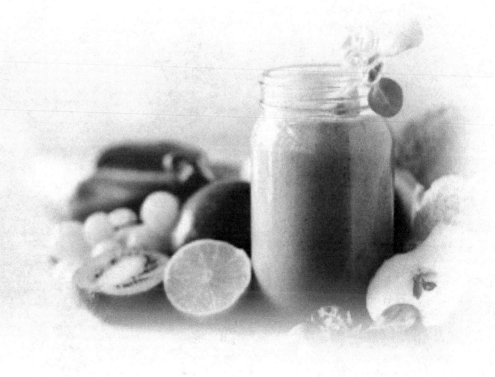

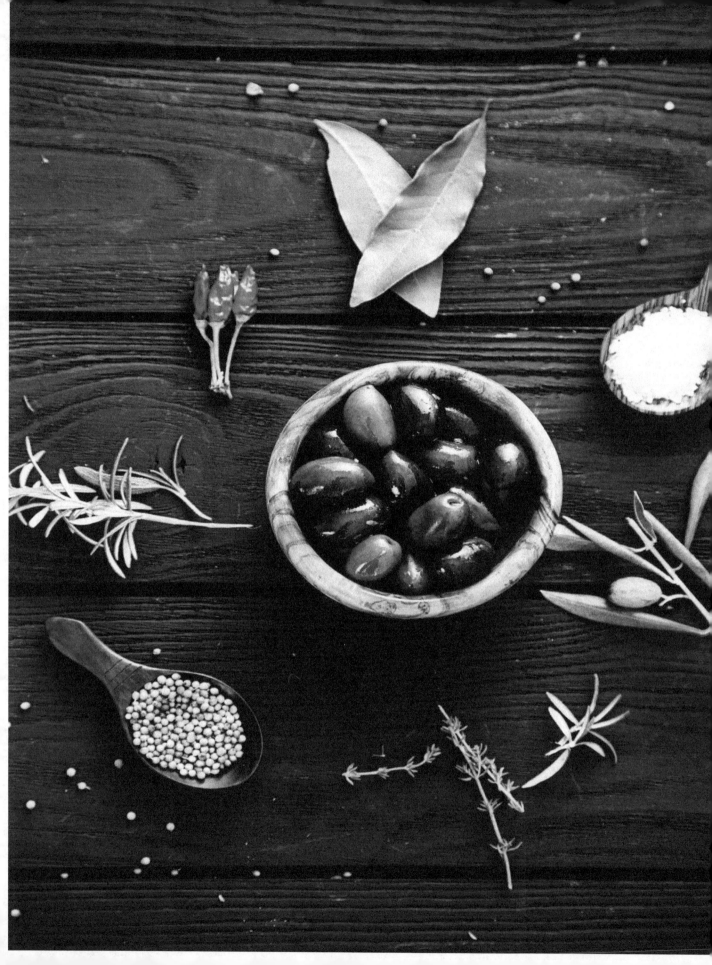

Introduction

The alkaline diet is based on a partial or complete exclusion of "acidic" foods.

Why should the alkaline diet help your body?

Scientists know that some foods form alkaline waste after digestion and others turn into acidic toxins. Scientists have found that cancer cells are particularly active in acidic environments: if there are too many acids, they tend to accumulate in the body and unbalance the acid-base balance: this can lead to the development of various diseases and acceleration of aging processes. The human body has a physiological tendency to oxidize; in order to function well, the body needs to maintain a perfect acid-base balance in the blood and tissues. Even a small deviation from the normal acid-base balance (7.35 - 7.45) can lead to serious problems. However, you can control this balance with a few but consistent habits: eat only alkaline foods! If you're a beginner, you can start by simply choosing more alkalizing foods in your daily menu and reducing those that increase acidity. The alkaline diet is not new: the benefits of this diet were demonstrated by Otto Barburg in 1932. However, the age of technology contributed to the foundation of this diet when it became a trend in 2018. Thankfully, one of the healthiest trends in recent years!

How does the alkaline diet help?

The alkaline diet is based on one simple law: do not eat foods considered acidic or acidic. Doing this, the body can produce the right amount of acidic metabolic wastes avoiding the accumulation of acids in the body and maintaining the body's natural pH levels.

Mains Acid-Forming Foods

- ✓ Coffee
- ✓ Red Meat
- ✓ Fish
- ✓ Light meat
- ✓ Cornmeal, Corn
- ✓ Rice
- ✓ Wheat Germ
- ✓ Cheese
- ✓ Mais
- ✓ Alcoholic drinks
- ✓ All sauces
- ✓ White flour
- ✓ Refined sugar
- ✓ Refined salt
- ✓ White vinegar
- ✓ Nutmeg

Main Alkalinizing Foods

- ✓ Peas
- ✓ Beans
- ✓ Grains: flax, millet, quinoa, and amaranth
- ✓ Potatoes
- ✓ Almonds, peanuts and nuts
- ✓ Coconut
- ✓ Fresh unsalted butter
- ✓ Raw yogurt
- ✓ Natural Fruit juices
- ✓ All vegetable juices
- ✓ Herbal teas
- ✓ Garlic
- ✓ Cayenne pepper
- ✓ Most herbs dressing
- ✓ All vegetables
- ✓ Unprocessed sea salt
- ✓ Raw honey
- ✓ Dried sugar cane

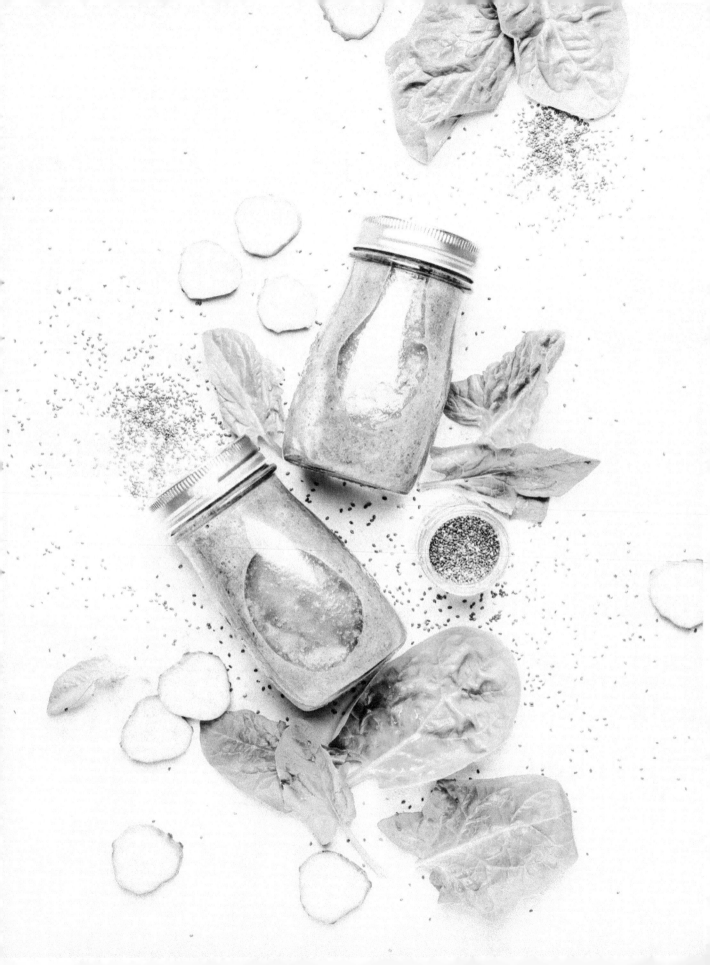

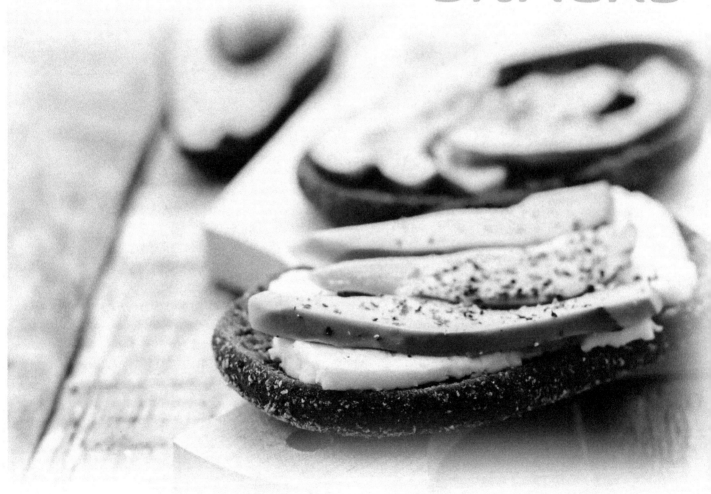

Chapter 1.
BREAKFAST AND
SNACKS

1) COBBLER OF CHIA SEEDS AND BLUEBERRIES

		Servings: 4

Ingredients:

- ✓ Blueberry Blend -
- ✓ Chia seeds, 1 tablespoon
- ✓ Unrefined whole cane sugar, 2 tablespoons
- ✓ Blueberries, 2 c.
- ✓ Topping -
- ✓ Almond flour, .5 c.
- ✓ Sea salt, .25 teaspoon
- ✓ Vanilla bean powder, 1 teaspoon

Ingredients:

- ✓ A mixture of baking soda and cream of tartar, 1.5 teaspoons
- ✓ Unrefined whole cane sugar, 2 tablespoons
- ✓ Melted coconut oil, 2 tablespoons
- ✓ Coconut milk, 4 tablespoons
- ✓ Oatmeal, .5 c.

Directions:

- ❖ Start by setting your oven to 350.
- ❖ To make the blueberries, mix the chia seeds, sugar and blueberries. Place blueberry mixture in the bottom of four 4-ounce baking cups.
- ❖ To fix the topping, mix together the salt, vanilla bean powder, baking powder, sugar, coconut oil, coconut milk, oatmeal and almond flour.

- ❖ Divide the blueberry topping among the four ramekins. You can leave the topping as spoonfuls, or you can spread it evenly over the blueberry mixture to create a full crust.
- ❖ Bake the cobblers for 45 minutes, or until the topping has turned golden brown and everything is heated through. Enjoy.

2) QUICK AND EASY GRANOLA BARS

		Servings: 6

Ingredients:

- ✓ Vanilla bean powder, .25 teaspoon
- ✓ Cinnamon spice, .25 teaspoon
- ✓ Sea salt, .25 teaspoon
- ✓ Coconut oil, 1 tablespoon

Ingredients:

- ✓ Brown rice syrup, 2 tablespoons
- ✓ Almond butter, .5 c.
- ✓ Quick rolled oats, 1 c.

Directions:

- ❖ Place some parchment in the bottom of a 9x5 inch baking dish.
- ❖ Add the vanilla bean powder, cinnamon, salt, coconut oil, brown rice syrup, almond butter and oats to a food processor and blend until well combined.

- ❖ Run the concoction into the loaf pan and push it down into an even dough, making sure it is firmly compressed. Refrigerate the bars for 15-20 minutes, or until completely firm.
- ❖ Cut granola into six bars and enjoy. Store leftovers in the refrigerator. At room temperature, they will become soft.

3) ALKALINE BLUEBERRY SPELT PANCAKES

Preparation Time: 6 mnutes.	**Cooking Time**: 20 minutes.	**Servings: 3**

Ingredients:

- ✓ 2 cups of spelt flour
- ✓ 1 cup coconut Milk
- ✓ 1/2 cup Alkaline Water
- ✓ 2 tbsps. Grape sed Oil

Ingredients:

- ✓ 1/2 cup Agave
- ✓ 1/2 cup Blueberries
- ✓ 1/4 teaspoon of musk Sea

Directions:

- ❖ Mix together in a beater the spellate flower, agave, wheat seed oil, hemp seeds and moss5s together.
- ❖ To the menstrual, add 1 cup of sheep's milk and cologne until you get the consistency menstrual you like.

- ❖ Mash the blue into the batter.
- ❖ Heat over medium heat and then lightly coat with the grain oil.
- ❖ Put the butter in the oven and let it cook for about 5 minutes on all sides.
- ❖ Serve and have fun.

4) ALKALINE BLUEBERRY MUFFINS

Preparation Time: 5 Minutes.	Cooking Time: 20 minutes.	Servings: 3

Ingredients:

- ✓ 1 cup of coconut milk
- ✓ 3/4 cup of Spelt Flour
- ✓ 3/4 Teff of flour
- ✓ 1/2 cup Blueberries

Ingredients:

- ✓ 1/3 cup of Agave
- ✓ 1/4 cup Sea Moss Gel
- ✓ 1/2 teaspoon coarse salt, ground salt, olive oil

Directions:

- ❖ Adjust the oven temperature to 365 degrees.
- ❖ Grate 6 regular-size muffin cups with muffin liners.
- ❖ In a bowl, mix together sea salt, se moss, agave, coconut milk, and flour gel until they are eproperly blnded.

- ❖ You then crimp in blueberries.
- ❖ Lightly cover the muffins with the wheat seed.
- ❖ Pour in the batter of muffin.
- ❖ Bake for at least 30 minutes until brown.
- ❖ Serve.

---

5) MEAL OF CRISPY QUINOA

Preparation Time: 5 minutes	Cooking Time: 25 minutes.	Servings: 2

Ingredients:

- ✓ 3 cups coco nut milk
- ✓ 1 cup rinsed quinoa.
- ✓ 1/8 tsp. cinnamon powder

Ingredients:

- ✓ 1 cup raspberry
- ✓ 1/2 coconut

Directions:

- ❖ In a saucepan, your milk and bring to a boil over moderate heat.
- ❖ Add the milk to the milk and then bring it to soak once more.
- ❖ Then let sit for at least 15 minutes over medium heat until the milk has reduced.

- ❖ Stand higher in the corner than in the middle of the world.
- ❖ Cook for 8 minutes until milk is ready to use.
- ❖ Add the raspberry and coook the meal for 30 seconds.
- ❖ Serve enjoy.

---

6) COCONUT PANCAKES

Preparation Time: 5 minutes.	Cooking Time: 15 minutes.	Servings: 4

Ingredients:

- ✓ 1 cup coconut flour
- ✓ 2 tbsps. Arrow root powder
- ✓ 1 tsp. baking powder

Ingredients:

- ✓ 1 cup coco walnut milk
- ✓ 3 tbsps. Coconut oil

Directions:

- ❖ In a medium container, mix all ingredients together.
- ❖ Add the coconut milk and 2 tbsps. Del coconut oil and mix properly.
- ❖ In a skillet, melt 1 tsp. of coco walnut oil.
- ❖ Pour a ladleful of batter inside the container and then spread the batter evenly over a smooth surface.

- ❖ Coook il form for a least 3 minutes on average heat until you becomes firm.
- ❖ Flip the pancake to the other side and then cook for another 2 minutes until golden brown.
- ❖ Cook the pancakes in a microwave oven.
- ❖ Serve.

7) QUINOA PORRIDGE

Preparation Time: 5 minutes.	Cooking Time: 25 minutes.	Servings: 2

✓ 2 cups coco nut milk
✓ 1 cup rinsed quinoa.

✓ 1/8 tsp. ground cinnamon
✓ 1 cup fresh blueberries

Directions:

❖ In a saucepan, boil the nut milk at a high temperature.
❖ Add the quinoa to the milk and then bring the mixture to a boil.
❖ Then you let it sit for 15 mnutes on medium heat until the milk has reduced.

❖ Add the cinnamon and then mix it properly in the refrigerator.
❖ Bake for at least 8 minutes until the milk is absorbed.
❖ Add the blue and light blue and then mix for another 30 seconds.
❖ Serve.

8) AMARANTH PORRIDGE

Preparation Time: 5 minutes.	Cooking Time: 30 minutes.	Servings: 2

✓ 2 cups coconut milk
✓ 2 cups alkaline water
✓ 1 cup of administrator

✓ 2 tbsps. Coconut oil
✓ 1 tbsp. land cinnamon

Directions:

❖ In a bowl, mix the milk with the water and then boil the milk.

❖ You put the amaranth in and then reduce the heat and make milk.

9) BANANA BARLEY PORRIDGE

Preparation Time: 15 minutes.	Cooking Time: 5 minutes.	Servings: 2

✓ 1 glass divided unsweetened coconut milk
✓ 1 small bernard cut into slices
✓ 1/2 cup barley

✓ 3 drops liquid stevia.
✓ 1/4 cup chopped coconuts

Directions:

❖ In a bowl, properly mix barley with half the coconut milk and stevia.
❖ Cover the bowl and let sit for about 6 hours.

❖ In a saucepan, mix the barley mixture with the coconut milk.
❖ Coook for about 5 minutes on moderate heat.
❖ Then top with chopped walnut and bernard.
❖ Serve.

10) ZUCCHINI MUFFINS

Preparation Time: 10 minutes.	Cooking Time: 25 minutes.	Servings: 16

✓ 1 tbsp. ground flaxsed
✓ 3 tbsps. Alkaline water
✓ 1/4 inch walnut
✓ 3 medium over-ripe banas
✓ 2 small grated zucchinis

✓ 1/2 cup coco walnut milk
✓ 1 tsp. vanilla extract
✓ 2 cups coconut flour
✓ 1 tbsp. baking powder
✓ 1 teaspoon of cinnamon 1/4 teaspoon of sea salt

Directions:

❖ Adjust the temperature of your oven to 375ºF.
❖ Grate the muffler tray with the appropriate cover.
❖ In a bowl, mix the flaxsed with the water.

❖ In a glass tumbler, massh the bananas and remaining ingredients.
❖ Mix thoroughly and then divide the mixture into the muffin molds.
❖ Bake for 25 minutes.
❖ Serve.

11) MILE PORRIDGE

Preparation Time: 10 minutes.	Cooking Time: 20 minutes.	Servings: 2

Ingredients:

- ✓ Sea salt
- ✓ 1 tbsp. finely chopped coconuts.
- ✓ 1/2 cup unsweetened coconut milk

Ingredients:

- ✓ 1/2 cup of millet rinsed and draned millet
- ✓ 1-1/2 cups water alkaline
- ✓ 3 Drops liquid stevia
- ❖ Cook for about 15 minutes, then add remaining ingredients. Stylize.
- ❖ Coook the meal for another 4 minutes.
- ❖ Serve the meal with a garnish of hazelnuts chopped.

Directions:

- ❖ Sauté the millet in a non-stick skillet for about 3 minutes.
- ❖ Add salt and water, then stir.
- ❖ Allow the meal to rest and reduce the amount of salt.

12) JACKFRUIT FRY VEGETABLE

Preparation Time: 5 minutes.	Cooking Time: 5 minutes.	Servings: 6

Ingredients:

- ✓ 2 onions small finely chopped
- ✓ 2 cups tomatoes chopped cherry finely
- ✓ 1/8 tablespoon of cassava butter
- ✓ 1 tablespoon olive oil

Ingredients:

- ✓ 2 seeded and chopped red bell peppers
- ✓ 3 cups firm jackfruit with seeds and chopped
- ✓ 1/8 teaspoon cayenne pepper
- ✓ 2 tbsps. Chopped fresh basil leaves Salt
- ❖ Then add the juice, pepper, salt and turmeric.
- ❖ Bake for about 8 minutes.
- ❖ Garnish the meal with basil leaves.
- ❖ Serve hot.

Directions:

- ❖ In a fat skillet, saute onions and bell peppers for about 5 minutes.
- ❖ Add tomatoes and stir.
- ❖ Coook for 2 minutes.

13) ZUCCHINI PANCAKES

Preparation Time: 15 minutes.	Cooking Time: 8 minutes.	Servings: 8

Ingredients:

- ✓ 12 tablespoons of alkaline water
- ✓ 6 great zucchini grateds
- ✓ Sea salt
- ✓ 4 tablespoons of Flax Seeds minced

Ingredients:

- ✓ 2 tsps. Olive oil
- ✓ 2 jalapeño peppers finely chopped
- ✓ 1/2 cup finely chopped scallions
- ❖ Add the flax and scallion mixture and then stir everything together.
- ❖ Preheat a grill and then grease it thoroughly with oil.
- ❖ Pour 1/4 zuchini mixture into a griddle and bake for 3 minutes.
- ❖ Flip the side carefully then coook for 2 more minutes.
- ❖ Repeat the procedure with the rest of the mass in random order.
- ❖ Serve.

Directions:

- ❖ In a bowl, mix together the water and flax and then set aside.
- ❖ Place our food in a large non-stick container and then place in a cooking container.
- ❖ Add the glass of milk, the glass of wine, and the glass of pumpkin.
- ❖ Cook for 3 minutes then transfer the zucchini into a boglio large.

14) SQUASH HASH

Preparation Time: 2 mnutes.	Cooking Time: 10 minutes.	Servings: 2

✓ 1 tsp. onion powder. ✓ 1/2 cup finely chopped onion	✓ 2 cups of spaghetti squash ✓ 1/2 teaspoon of sea salt

Directions: ❖ Using paper towels, squeze extra moisture from spaghetti squash. ❖ Place the squash in a bowl, then add the salt, onion and onion powder. ❖ Stir well to mix it up. ❖ Spray a non-stick cooking skillet with cooooking spray that place il over moderate heat.	❖ Add the spaghetti squash. ❖ Coook the squash for 5 minutes. ❖ Fluff up the browns with a spatula. ❖ Coook formatis of 5 minutes until the crispness is reached desired. ❖ Serve.

15) HEMP SEED PORRIDGE

Preparation Time: 5 minutes.	Cooking Time: 5 minutes.	Servings: 6

✓ 3 cups cooked hemp sed ✓ 1 packet Stevia	✓ 1 cup coco of walnut milk

Directions: ❖ In a bowl, mix the milk and nut milk for about 5 minutes. ❖ Remove the pan from the heat and add the stevia. Stylize.	❖ Serve in 6 bowls. ❖ Enjoy.

16) VEGGIE MEDLEY

Preparation Time: 5 mnutes.	Cooking Time: 10 minutes.	Servings: 2

✓ 1 seed and a bacon ✓ 1/2 cup lime juice ✓ 2 tablespoons of fresh cilantro ✓ 1/2 tsp. cumin ✓ 1 teaspoon of sea salt ✓ 1 wooden jacket	✓ 1/2 cup zucchini ✓ 1 cup halved cherry tomatoes ✓ 1/2 cup sliced mushrooms ✓ 1 cup coooked broccoli florets ✓ 1 sweet onion chopped

Directions: ❖ Spray a dab of paint with stick pan with cooking spray and then place it all over the body. ❖ Add the butter, tomatoes, chili, grapes, pumpkin, peanut butter and mushroms.	❖ Cook for about 7 minutes as you stir from time to time. ❖ Add the cumin and caraway and then the pepper. ❖ Cook for an additional 3 minutes while stirring. ❖ Heat the pan from the heat and add the lime juice. ❖ Serve.

17) PUMPKIN SPICE QUINOA

Preparation Time: 10 minutes.	Cooking Time: 0 minutes.	Servings: 2

✓ 1 cup of cooked quinoa ✓ 1 cup unsweetened coconut milk ✓ 1 large mashed banana	✓ 1/4 cup pumpkin pureee ✓ 1 tsp. pumpkin spice ✓ 2 teaspoons of chia seds

Directions: ❖ In a container, mix all ingredients together. ❖ Close the lid and then close the container so that it mixes.	❖ Refrigerate overnight. ❖ Serve.

Chapter 2. LUNCH

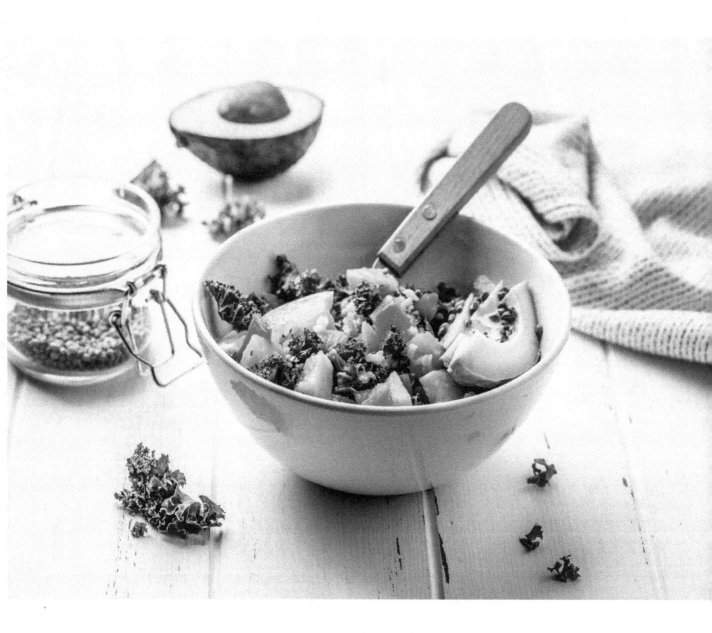

18) KAMUT PATTIES

Preparation Time: 15 minutes.	Cooking Time: 30 minutes.	Servings: 3-4

✓ 3 cups of cooked Kamut Cereal	✓ ½ teaspoon of Cayenne Powder
✓ 1 cup of chopped Red Onions	✓ 1 tablespoon of Oregano
✓ 1 cup of green peppers and Yellow chopped	✓ 1 tablespoon of Onion Powder.
✓ 1 cup of Spelt Flour	✓ 1 teaspoon of salt Pure Sea
✓ ½ cup of Homemade Hempseed Milk	✓ 2 tablespoons of Grade Seed Oil
✓ 1 tablespoon of Basil	

Directions:

❖ Cook patties for about 4 or 5 minutes on each side.
❖ Serve and enjoy your kamut meatballs!
❖ Tips useful:
❖ If you don't have Spelt flour, add Gärbazo Bean Flour instead flour.
❖ You can enjoy kamut meatballs with our "Cheese" French or French Tomato Sauce.

❖ Combine the vegetables, hemp seed milk, hemp seed flour and kamut milk in a large bowl.
❖ Place 1/2 cup of spelt flour in the bowl and mix well. Keep adding more flour until you can form a patties shape.
❖ Heat soybean oil in a skillet over medium heat. Form patties from the mixture and place in the oven.

19) MUSHROOM BURGERS PORTOBELLO

Preparation Time: 25 minutes.	Cooking Time: 50 Minutes.	Servings: 2

✓ 2 cups of Portobello Mushrom caps	✓ 1/2 teaspoon of Cayenne
✓ 1 sliced Avocado	✓ 1 teaspoon of Oregano.
✓ 1 sliced Plum Tomatoes	✓ 2 teaspoons of Basil
✓ 1 cup of torn Lettuce	✓ 3 tablespoons of olive oil
✓ 1 cup of Purslane	

Directions:

❖ Lay out the mushrom cap on a serving dish. This will serve as the basis for the Mushroom Burger.
❖ On it are avocado, tomatoes, lettuce and puree.
❖ Cover the burger with another mushroom capm. Repeat step 7 and 8 with the mushrooms and vermicelli.
❖ Feel and enjoy our Portobello Mushroom Burgers!
❖ Useful Tips:
❖ You can add any type of lettuce, exotic lettuce, chives and other ingredients depending on your taste.
❖ You can serve Portobello Mushroom Burgers with our "Chese" Sauce or Fragrant Tomato Sauce.

❖ Preheat your oven at 425 degrees Fahrenheit.
❖ Remove the mushroom and cut 1/2 inch off the top slice, as if you were slicing a sandwich.
❖ In a medium bowl mix the alder powder, cinnamon, oregano, olive oil and butter.
❖ Cover a sheet of baking paper with the sheet and brush with the grape oil to prevent sticking.
❖ Place mushroom caps on baking sheet and brush with prepared marinade. Marinate for 10 minutes before baking begins.
❖ Bake for 10 minutes until brown, then unmold. Continue to bake for another 10 minutes.

20) HEALTHY FRIED-RICE

Preparation Time: 15 minutes.	Cooking Time: 50 minutes.	Servings: 2

✓ 1 cup of cooked Wild Rice	✓ 1/4 onion, diced
✓ 1/2 cup of sliced Mushrooms	✓ Pure Sea Salt, a taste
✓ 1/2 cup of cubed Zucchini	✓ Cayenne Powder, per taste
✓ 1/2 cup of cubed Bell Peppers	✓ 1/2 tablespoon of Grape Seed Oil

Directions:

❖ Add the Wild Rice boiled to the oven and continue to process until lightly browned.
❖ Serve and enjoy your Healthy Fried-Rice!
❖ Useful Tips:
❖ If you want, you can use cooked quinoa instead.

❖ Heat soybean oil in a medium skillet over medium heat.
❖ Add the onion diced to the skillet and sauté until golden brown.
❖ Add the mushrooms, Zucchini and Peppers bell and coook for 5 more minutes. The vegetables should get a little softer.

21) VEG-MEATBALLS

Preparation Time: 10 minutes.	**Cooking Time**: 30 minutes	**Servings**: 7-9

Ingredients:

- ✓ 1 1/2 cups of Garbanzo Beans cooked
- ✓ 1 cup of Garbanzo Bean Flour
- ✓ 2 cups of Mushrooms
- ✓ 1/4 cup of diced Green Peppers
- ✓ 1/2 cup of diced Onions
- ✓ 2 teaspoons of Oregano
- ✓ 1 tablespoon of Onion Powder
- ✓ 2 teaspoons of Basil
- ✓ 1 teaspoon of Fennel Powder

Ingredients:

- ✓ 1 teaspoon of Dill
- ✓ 1 teaspoon of Savory
- ✓ 1 teaspoon of Sage
- ✓ 1/2 teaspoon of Ginger Powder 1/2 teaspoon of Ground Cloves
- ✓ 1 teaspoon of Pure Sea Salt
- ✓ 1/2 teaspoon of cayenne powder
- ✓ 6 cups by Fragrant Tomato Sauce
- ✓ 2 tablespoons or semi-fat oil

Directions:

- ❖ Place the cooked mushrooms, Garbanzo beans, onions, green peppers and seasonings into a processor. Blend well for 1 minute.
- ❖ Add the dough to a large bowl and mix with Garrbazo Bean Flour. Cut into a ball of dough. If they do not form, add more sugar.
- ❖ Turn off the meatballs and let them rest for a couple minutes.
- ❖ Add Grape Seed Oil to a pot and heat over low heat.

- ❖ Place a couple of patties on the pan. Bake for 2 minutes on each side.
- ❖ Add Fragrant Tomato Sauce to the meatballs and simmer for 5 minutes.
- ❖ Serve and enjoy your Meatballs!
- ❖ Useful Tips:
- ❖ You can use it with our flat bread or Homemade bread dough.

22) ROASTED ARTICHOKE SALAD

		Servings: 2

- ✓ Paprika, pinch
- ✓ Garlic powder, a pinch
- ✓ Pepper, pinch
- ✓ Sea salt, a pinch
- ✓ Avocado oil, 1 tablespoon
- ✓ Drained artichoke hearts, 14 ounces
- ✓ Mixed salad, 2-4 c.

- ✓ Seasoning -
- ✓ Pepper, pinch
- ✓ Sea salt, a pinch
- ✓ Shallot diced
- ✓ Brown rice sweetener, 1 tablespoon
- ✓ Sesame seeds, 1 tablespoon
- ✓ Apple vinegar, 2 tablespoons
- ✓ Avocado oil, 2 tablespoons

Directions:

- ❖ Start by setting your oven to 425. Place some parchment on a baking sheet.
- ❖ Cut off the tips of the artichokes and then cut the hearts in half. Rub them with a little oil.
- ❖ Stir in paprika, garlic, pepper and salt. Arrange the artichokes on the baking sheet and sprinkle with the seasoning mixture. Stir to coat.

- ❖ Roast them for 30 minutes, tossing again halfway through the cooking time.
- ❖ While the artichokes are roasting, whisk together the pepper, salt, shallots, brown rice syrup, sesame seeds, vinegar and avocado oil. Make sure everything is well mixed. Adjust the flavors as needed.
- ❖ To assemble the salad, toss the salad mix with the artichokes and then pour in the dressing. Divide between two plates and enjoy.

23) ARTICHOKE HASH

		Servings: 4

- ✓ Sliced shallot
- ✓ EVOO
- ✓ Pepper

- ✓ Halls
- ✓ Brussels sprouts thinly sliced, 6
- ✓ Sliced mushrooms, 4

Directions:

- ❖ Pour cold water into a bowl.
- ❖ Place the sliced artichokes in the water and let them rest.
- ❖ Rinse well and pat dry with paper towels.
- ❖ Place a skillet on medium and heat a little EVOO.

- ❖ Add the artichokes and Brussels sprouts. Cook for four minutes.
- ❖ Sprinkle with pepper and salt.
- ❖ Serve with a drizzle of olive oil and sprinkle with sliced scallions

24) VEGETABLE FRITTERS

Servings: 2

Ingredients:

- ✓ Kitchen spray
- ✓ Water, .25 c.
- ✓ Garlic powder, .5 tsp
- ✓ Salt, 1 teaspoon
- ✓ Almond flour, .25 c.

Directions:

- ❖ Place shallots, almond flour, yellow squash, zucchini, carrot, garlic powder and salt in a food processor.
- ❖ Pulse until everything is completely mixed.
- ❖ Add just enough water to make sure the mixture is moist and thick.

Ingredients:

- ✓ Shallots, 4
- ✓ Grated onion, .5
- ✓ Chopped yellow pumpkin, 1
- ✓ Peeled and chopped carrot, 1
- ✓ Chopped zucchini, 1

- ❖ Place a large skillet over standard heat and spray with prep spray.
- ❖ When the oil is heated, use an ice cream scoop and add the mixture to the pan. Cook for three minutes per side.
- ❖ Use the back of the ice cream scoop to spread the mixture.

25) MINT AND LIME SALAD

Servings: 4

Ingredients:

- ✓ Lemon juice, 2 tablespoons
- ✓ Chopped mint, 2 tablespoons
- ✓ Strawberries, .25 c.
- ✓ Diced peaches, .25 c.
- ✓ Mandarin segments, .25 c.

Directions:

- ❖ Place all the fruit in a bowl. Add the mint and lemon juice.

Ingredients:

- ✓ Pieces of chopped cantaloupe, .25 c.
- ✓ Bite-sized pieces of honeydew, .25 c.
- ✓ Bite-sized pieces of watermelon, .25 c.
- ✓ Diced apple, .25 c.
- ✓ Grapes, .25 c.

- ❖ Mix well and cover.
- ❖ Refrigerate and chill overnight.

26) ZUCCHINI SALAD

Servings: 2

Ingredients:

- ✓ Fresh herbs of your choice, 1 teaspoon
- ✓ Pepper
- ✓ Halls
- ✓ EVOO, 2 tablespoons
- ✓ Juice of 0,5 lemons

Directions:

- ❖ Wash all vegetables and set aside.
- ❖ Cut off the ends of the zucchini. Cut in half lengthwise and then slice into half moons.
- ❖ Dice the tomatoes.
- ❖ Cut the bell bell pepper in half, clean the ribs and seeds and slice each half.

Ingredients:

- ✓ Chopped garlic, 1 clove
- ✓ Sliced onion, 1
- ✓ Diced tomato, 2
- ✓ Red bell pepper, 1
- ✓ Sliced zucchini, 1

- ❖ Cut off top and bottom of onion and remove outer skin. Thinly slice into rings.
- ❖ Add all prepared vegetables to a bowl.
- ❖ In a separate bowl, add pepper, salt, herbs, olive oil, garlic and lemon juice. Mix well to combine.
- ❖ Pour over vegetables and stir to coat.

27) FRIED TOFU

Ingredients:

- ✓ Fresh herbs
- ✓ Ginger, .25 tablespoons
- ✓ Curry powder, .5 tablespoons
- ✓ Pepper
- ✓ Halls
- ✓ EVOO, 2 tablespoons
- ✓ Coconut milk, 1.5 c.
- ✓ Chopped green beans, .5 lb.

Ingredients:

- ✓ Diced bell pepper - green, bell, 1 piece
- ✓ Diced bell pepper - red, bell, 1 piece
- ✓ Diced tomatoes, 3
- ✓ Chopped zucchini, 3
- ✓ Diced firm tofu, 1 lb.

Directions:

- ❖ Place a saucepan on medium, heat the oil. Add the tofu and cook about three minutes.
- ❖ Add the zucchini, beans and peppers. Sauté for an additional three minutes.

- ❖ Add the tomatoes and coconut milk and mix well. Allow to simmer for a little longer.
- ❖ Season with herbs, curry powder, pepper, salt and ginger.
- ❖ Serve with wild rice.

28) POTATO AND PUMPKIN MEATBALLS

Servings: 2

Ingredients:

- ✓ EVOO
- ✓ Pepper
- ✓ Halls
- ✓ Chopped parsley, 3 tablespoons

Ingredients:

- ✓ Water, 4 tablespoons
- ✓ Soybean flour, 2.5 ounces
- ✓ Potatoes, 1 lb.
- ✓ Pumpkin, 1 lb.

Directions:

- ❖ Peel the potatoes and squash. Cut them into large pieces.
- ❖ Place in a food processor and process until small pieces but not mush.
- ❖ Add the water and soy flour to a bowl. Stir well.
- ❖ Remove the squash and potato from the food processor and place them in another bowl.

- ❖ Pour over flour mixture and mix well.
- ❖ Season with pepper, parsley and salt.
- ❖ Place a skillet over medium heat and heat a little EVOO.
- ❖ Turn the potato and pumpkin mixture into meatballs. Place the prepared patties in the skillet and fry for three minutes per side.

29) ITALIAN SOFFRITTO

Servings: 2

Ingredients:

- ✓ Water, .5 c
- ✓ Pepper
- ✓ Curry powder, .5 teaspoons
- ✓ Oregano plant, 1 teaspoon
- ✓ Parsley, one tablespoon
- ✓ Sodium chloride, 1 teaspoon

Ingredients:

- ✓ Grated cheddar, 1 tablespoon
- ✓ EVOO, 2 tablespoons
- ✓ Diced tomatoes, 2
- ✓ Zucchini flakes, 1
- ✓ Diced onion, 2
- ✓ Leeks in flakes, 2

Directions:

- ❖ Take a frying pan and heat the olive oil.
- ❖ Place the onions in the skillet and cook until soft.
- ❖ Add the zucchini and cook an additional four minutes. Pour the water into the pan and put a lid on.
- ❖ Lower the heat and simmer for ten minutes.

- ❖ Carefully remove the lid and add the tomatoes. Season with curry powder and pepper. Replace the lid and cook another ten minutes.
- ❖ When cooked, taste and adjust seasonings if necessary.
- ❖ Sprinkle with cheese and serve with bread if your diet permits.

30) SOUTHERN SALAD

		Servings: 4

✓ Sauce, .5 c.	✓ Halved cherry tomatoes, 1 c.
✓ Cilantro, .5 c.	✓ Sprouted black beans, .5 c.
✓ Chopped almonds, .25 c.	✓ Romaine lettuce, 5 c.
✓ Diced avocado, 1	

Directions:

❖ Divide among salad bowls and serve.

❖ Place each content in an oversized bowl and toss well.

31) ROASTED VEGETABLES

		Servings: 4

✓ Halls	✓ Chopped carrot, one
✓ Allium (garlic) powder, 1 tablespoon	✓ Cut asparagus, .5 bunch
✓ Coconut oil, 1 tablespoon	✓ Cherry tomatoes, 1 pint
✓ Pepper - crushed, bell yellow, one	✓ Halved mushrooms, .5 c.
✓ Pepper - crushed, bell red, one	

Directions:

❖ Pass over the vegetables and toss to coat.
❖ Pour the vegetables onto a kitchen wrap then place on the stove for 15 minutes until the vegetables are tender.
❖ Divide among four plates and enjoy.

❖ You need to heat the oven to 425.
❖ Place the carrot, peppers, tomatoes, mushrooms and asparagus in a large bowl.
❖ In another bowl, place the garlic powder, sodium chloride and coconut milk. Mix well.

32) PAD THAI SALAD

		Servings: 2

✓ Salt, .5 tsp	✓ Chopped shallot, 1
✓ Stevia, 1 packet	✓ Peeled zucchini, 1
✓ Tamarind paste, 1 teaspoon	✓ Thinly sliced carrot, 2
✓ Chopped garlic, 1 clove	✓ Bean sprouts, 1 c.
✓ Juice of a lime	✓ Iceberg lettuce, 4 c.
✓ Chopped almonds, 2 tablespoons	

❖ Place the almonds, bean sprouts, zucchini, carrots and lettuce in a large bowl.
❖ Place the salt, stevia, lime juice, tamarind paste and garlic in a small food processor. Process until well blended.

❖ Pour the dressing over the vegetables and toss to coat.
❖ Divide evenly among serving bowls.

33) CUCUMBER SALAD

		Servings: 4

✓ Pepper	✓ Chopped garlic, 4 cloves
✓ Halls	✓ Cucumber, 1 lb.
✓ Sesame seed oil, 3 tablespoons	

❖ Place the pepper, salt, sesame seed oil and garlic in a bowl. Whisk well to combine. Wash the cucumbers and cut off the ends.

❖ Cut them in half lengthwise and then slice them into half moons.
❖ Add the dressing mixture to the cucumbers and toss well to coat.
❖ Place in the refrigerator for ten minutes. Enjoy.

34) PASTA SALAD WITH RED LENTILS

		Servings: 4

✓ For the dressing and pasta - ✓ Pepper, .25 tsp ✓ Sea salt, .25 tsp ✓ Dried oregano, 1 teaspoon ✓ Lemon juice, one tablespoon ✓ Apple vinegar, two tablespoons ✓ Avocado - oil, .25 c. ✓ Red lentil pasta, 2 c.	✓ Vegetables - ✓ Crushed garlic, 2 cloves ✓ Sliced summer squash, .5 ✓ Sliced zucchini, .5 ✓ Diced red onion, .33 c. ✓ Chopped bell pepper - orange, bell, 1 c. ✓ Chopped asparagus stems, 6 ✓ Avocado oil, 1 tablespoon

Directions:

❖ Cook the pasta according to the directions on the package.

❖ While the pasta is cooking, whisk together the pepper, salt, oregano, lemon juice, vinegar and avocado oil until well combined. Adjust any seasoning that you need.

❖ For the vegetables, heat the oil in an oversized skillet and cook the garlic, squash, zucchini, onion, bell bell pepper and asparagus. Cook for two to three minutes, or until soft.

❖ Add the pasta, vegetables and dressing to a bowl and toss to combine. Divide among four plates and enjoy.

35) SALAD WITH PEACH SAUCE

		Servings: 2

Ingredients:

✓ Seasoning -
✓ Pinch of sea salt
✓ Lemon juice, 1 teaspoon
✓ Water, .25 c
✓ Brown rice syrup, 3 to 4 tablespoons
✓ Tahini, 4 tablespoons
✓ Sauce -
✓ Diced Jalapeno, .5

Ingredients:

✓ Chopped purple onion, one tablespoon
✓ Diced coriander, one tablespoon
✓ Chopped bell pepper - red, bell, .25 c.
✓ Peach cubed and pitted
✓ Assembly -
✓ Mixed green salad - 3 c

Directions:

❖ For the dressing, whisk together the salt, lemon juice, water, brown rice syrup and tahini until combined. Adjust the seasonings as you need them.

❖ Toss each of the dressing ingredients inside another container.

❖ To make the salad, place the green salad on two plates and cover with the dressing. Drizzle with the dressing and enjoy.

36) PINEAPPLE SALAD

		Servings: 1

✓ Seasoning - ✓ Chopped cilantro, .5 c. ✓ Chopped shallots, .5 c. ✓ Lime juice, 2 tablespoons ✓ Water, .25 c. ✓ Avocado oil, .25 c. ✓ Sea salt, 0.5 teaspoons	✓ Garlic, 2 cloves ✓ Assembly - ✓ Dulce flakes ✓ Chopped purple cabbage, 1 c. ✓ Cubed pineapple, .5 c. ✓ Mixed salad, 2 c.

Directions:

❖ Place each seasoning content in your blender and blend until well combined. Adjust the seasonings as needed.

❖ To make the salad, add the green salad to a bowl and add the dulse flakes, purple cabbage and pineapple. Pour in the dressing and toss to combine. Enjoy.

37) SWEET POTATO SALAD WITH JALAPENO SAUCE

Servings: 2

Ingredients:

- ✓ Sweet potatoes -
- ✓ Sea salt, .25 tsp
- ✓ Paprika, 1 teaspoon
- ✓ Crushed garlic, 2 cloves
- ✓ Avocado oil, 2 tablespoons
- ✓ Sweet potatoes peeled and diced, 3
- ✓ Seasoning -
- ✓ Water, 1 c.

Ingredients:

- ✓ Sea salt, 0.5 teaspoons
- ✓ Lime juice, 2 tablespoons
- ✓ Jalapeno
- ✓ Cilantro leaves, .25 c.
- ✓ Raw cashews, 1 c.
- ✓ Assembly -
- ✓ Mixed salad, 2 c.

Directions:

- ❖ Start by setting your kitchen appliance to three hundred and fifty degrees. Place some parchment on some kitchen foil.
- ❖ Cough up the diced sweet potatoes with the salt, paprika, garlic and avocado oil. Make sure the potatoes are well coated.

- ❖ Spread the sweet potatoes on the baking sheet and bake for 25 minutes, or until soft.
- ❖ While the potatoes are cooking, add the salt, lime juice, jalapeno, cilantro, cashews and water to a high-speed blender and blend until smooth.
- ❖ To make the salad, divide the green salad into two plates and top with the cooked sweet potatoes. Add the dressing and toss to combine.

38) ASPARAGUS SALAD WITH LEMON SAUCE

Ingredients:

- ✓ Salad -
- ✓ Pepper, .25 tsp
- ✓ Sea salt, 0.5 teaspoons
- ✓ Crushed garlic, 3 cloves
- ✓ Diced onion, .5 c.
- ✓ Diced asparagus stems, 24
- ✓ Avocado oil, 1 teaspoon

Ingredients:

- ✓ Seasoning -
- ✓ Pepper
- ✓ Sea salt, .25 tsp
- ✓ Lemon juice, 2 tablespoons
- ✓ Water, .5 c.
- ✓ Raw cashews, .5 c.
- ✓ Assembly -
- ✓ Mixed salad, 2 c.

Directions:

- ❖ For the asparagus, heat the oil in a massive skillet and put in the pepper, salt, garlic, onion bulb, then the asparagus. Prepare for five to seven minutes, or until the onion has become soft.
- ❖ To make the dressing, add half of the cooked asparagus mixture to a blender along with the pepper, salt, lemon juice, water and cashews.

- ❖ Blend until smooth and creamy.
- ❖ To make the salad, divide the vegetable mixture between two plates and top with the rest of the cooked asparagus. Top with the dressing and enjoy.

39) VEGETARIAN LETTUCE ROLLS

Preparation Time: 20 minutes	Cooking Time: 10 minutes	Servings: 4

Ingredients:

- ✓ For filling:
- ✓ 1 teaspoon of olive oil
- ✓ 2 cups fresh shiitake mushrooms, chopped
- ✓ 2 teaspoons of tamari, divided
- ✓ 1 cup of cooked quinoa
- ✓ 1 teaspoon fresh lime juice
- ✓ 1 teaspoon organic apple cider vinegar
- ✓ ¼ cup shallots, chopped
- ✓ Sea salt and freshly ground black pepper, to taste
- ✓ For the creamy sauce:
- ✓ 5 ounces of silken tofu, pressed, drained and chopped
- ✓ 1 small clove of garlic, minced

Ingredients:

- ✓ ¼ cup of plain almond butter
- ✓ 1 teaspoon fresh lime juice
- ✓ Sea salt and freshly ground black pepper, to taste
- ✓ For wrappers:
- ✓ 8 medium lettuce leaves
- ✓ ¼ cup cucumber, peeled and cut into julienne strips
- ✓ ¼ cup of carrot, peeled and cut into julienne strips
- ✓ ¼ cup of cabbage, shredded

Directions:

- ❖ For the filling in a skillet, heat oil over medium heat and cook mushrooms and 1 teaspoon tamari for about 5-8 minutes, stirring often.
- ❖ Stir in the quinoa, lime juice, vinegar and remaining tamari and cook for about 1 minute, stirring constantly.
- ❖ Add the shallot, salt and black pepper and immediately remove from heat.

- ❖ Set aside to cool.
- ❖ Meanwhile, for the sauce: in a food processor, add all ingredients and pulse until smooth.
- ❖ Arrange the lettuce leaves on serving plates.
- ❖ Place quinoa filling evenly on each leaf and top with cucumbers, carrots and cabbage.
- ❖ Serve alongside the creamy sauce.

40) OATMEAL, TOFU AND SPINACH BURGER

Preparation Time: 15 minutes	Cooking Time: 16 minutes	Servings: 4

Ingredients:

- ✓ 1 pound of firm tofu, drained, pressed and crumbled
- ✓ ¾ cup rolled oats
- ✓ ¼ cup of flaxseed
- ✓ 2 cups frozen kale, thawed, squeezed, and chopped
- ✓ 1 medium onion, finely chopped
- ✓ 4 cloves of garlic, minced

Ingredients:

- ✓ 1 teaspoon of ground cumin
- ✓ 1 teaspoon of red pepper flakes, crushed
- ✓ Sea salt and freshly ground black pepper, to taste
- ✓ 2 tablespoons of olive oil
- ✓ 6 cups of fresh salad

Directions:

- ❖ In a large bowl, add all ingredients except oil and green salads and mix until well combined.
- ❖ Set aside for about 10 minutes.
- ❖ Cut out patties of the desired size from the dough.

- ❖ In a nonstick skillet, heat oil over medium heat and cook patties for 6-8 minutes per side.
- ❖ Serve these patties alongside the green salad.

41) HAMBURGER WITH BEANS, NUTS AND VEGETABLES

Preparation Time: 20 minutes	Cooking Time: 25 minutes	Servings: 4

Ingredients:

- ✓ ½ cup of walnuts
- ✓ 1 carrot, peeled and chopped
- ✓ 1 celery stalk, chopped
- ✓ 4 shallots, chopped
- ✓ 5 cloves of garlic, minced
- ✓ 2¼ cups canned black beans, rinsed and drained

Ingredients:

- ✓ 2½ cups sweet potato, peeled and grated
- ✓ ½ teaspoon of red pepper flakes, crushed
- ✓ ¼ teaspoon cayenne pepper
- ✓ Sea salt and freshly ground black pepper, to taste
- ✓ 12 cups of fresh vegetables

Directions:

- ❖ Preheat oven to 400 degrees F. Line a baking sheet with baking paper.
- ❖ In a food processor, add the walnuts and pulse until finely ground.
- ❖ Add the carrot, celery, shallot and garlic and pulse until finely chopped.
- ❖ Transfer the vegetable mixture to a large bowl.
- ❖ In the same food processor, add the beans and pulse until chopped.
- ❖ Add 1 1/2 cups sweet potato and pulse until it forms a chunky mixture.

- ❖ Transfer the bean mixture to the bowl with the vegetable mixture.
- ❖ Stir in the remaining sweet potato, spices, salt and black pepper and mix until well combined.
- ❖ Make 8 equal-sized patties with the bean mixture.
- ❖ Arrange the meatballs on the prepared baking sheet in a single layer.
- ❖ Bake for about 25 minutes.
- ❖ Divide vegetables among serving plates and top each with 2 meatballs.
- ❖ Serve immediately.

42) AVOCADOS STUFFED WITH TOFU AND BROCCOLI

Preparation Time: 20 minutes	Cooking Time: 15 minutes	Servings: 6

Ingredients:

For the marinade:
- ✓ ¼ cup fresh parsley leaves, chopped
- ✓ 1 small clove of garlic chopped
- ✓ 1 teaspoon fresh lemon zest, finely grated
- ✓ 1 tablespoon Dijon mustard
- ✓ ¼ cup of olive oil
- ✓ 2 tablespoons fresh lemon juice
- ✓ ¼ teaspoon ground cumin
- ✓ Sea salt and freshly ground black pepper, to taste

Ingredients:

- ✓ 1 (8-ounce) package of solid tofu, drained, pressed and cut into ½-inch slices
- ✓ 1 cup of broccoli florets

For the stuffed avocados:
- ✓ 1 tablespoon fresh chives, chopped
- ✓ 3 firm avocados, peeled, halved and pitted
- ✓ Sea salt and freshly ground black pepper, to taste
- ✓ 2 tablespoons fresh parsley, chopped

Directions:

- ❖ For the marinade: in a large bowl, add all ingredients except the tofu and beat until well combined.
- ❖ Add the tofu and broccoli and top generously with the marinade.
- ❖ Cover the bowl and refrigerate for about 1 hour.
- ❖ Preheat grill to medium-high heat. Generously grease the grill grate.
- ❖ Place the tofu slices on the grill and cook for about 2 minutes per side.
- ❖ Grill the broccoli florets for about 8-10 minutes, turning occasionally.

- ❖ Remove the tofu and broccoli from the grill and transfer to a large bowl.
- ❖ Set aside to cool slightly.
- ❖ Next, cut the tofu and broccoli into small pieces.
- ❖ Transfer the tofu and broccoli to a bowl with the chives and mix well.
- ❖ Sprinkle avocado halves with salt and black pepper.
- ❖ Stuff each half evenly with the tofu mixture.
- ❖ Garnish with parsley and serve immediately.

Chapter 3.
DINNER

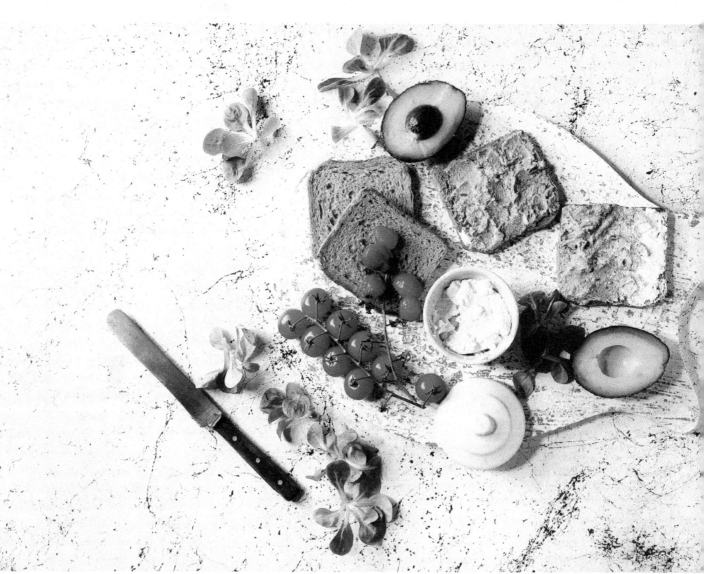

43) VEGETABLE SOUP

Preparation Time: 15 minutes	Cooking Time: 25 minutes	Servings: 3

Ingredients:

- ✓ ½ tablespoon of olive oil
- ✓ 2 tablespoons chopped onion
- ✓ 2 teaspoons of minced garlic
- ✓ ½ cup carrots, peeled and chopped
- ✓ ½ cup of green cabbage, chopped
- ✓ 1/3 cup French beans, crushed

Ingredients:

- ✓ 3 cups of homemade vegetable broth
- ✓ ½ tablespoon fresh lemon juice
- ✓ 3 tablespoons of water
- ✓ 2 tablespoons arrowroot starch
- ✓ Sea salt and freshly ground black pepper, to taste

Directions:

- ❖ Heat the oil in a large heavy-bottomed skillet over medium heat and sauté the onion and garlic for about 4-5 minutes.
- ❖ Add the carrots, cabbage and beans and cook for about 4-5 minutes, stirring often.
- ❖ Stir in the broth and bring to a boil.
- ❖ Cook for about 4-5 minutes.

- ❖ Meanwhile, in a small bowl, dissolve arrowroot starch in water.
- ❖ Slowly add the arrowroot starch mixture, stirring constantly.
- ❖ Cook for about 7-8 minutes, stirring occasionally.
- ❖ Add the lemon juice, salt and black pepper and remove from heat.
- ❖ Serve hot.

44) LENTIL AND SPINACH SOUP

Preparation Time: 15 minutes	Cooking Time: 1¼ hours. Total time: 1½ hoursPayments	Servings: 6

Ingredients:

- ✓ 2 tablespoons of olive oil
- ✓ 2 carrots, peeled and cut into pieces
- ✓ 2 stalks of celery, chopped
- ✓ 2 sweet onions, chopped
- ✓ 3 garlic cloves, minced
- ✓ 1½ cups brown lentils, rinsed
- ✓ 2 cups of tomatoes, finely chopped
- ✓ ¼ teaspoon dried basil, crushed
- ✓ ¼ teaspoon dried oregano, crushed
- ✓ ¼ teaspoon dried thyme, crushed

Ingredients:

- ✓ 1 teaspoon of ground cumin
- ✓ ½ teaspoon of ground coriander
- ✓ ½ teaspoon of paprika
- ✓ 6 cups of vegetable broth
- ✓ 3 cups fresh spinach, chopped
- ✓ Sea salt and freshly ground black pepper, to taste
- ✓ 2 tablespoons fresh lemon juice

Directions:

- ❖ In a large soup pot, heat the oil over medium heat and sauté the carrot, celery and onion for about 5 minutes.
- ❖ Add the garlic and sauté for about 1 minute.
- ❖ Add the lentils and sauté for about 3 minutes.
- ❖ Stir in the tomatoes, herbs, spices and broth and bring to a boil.

- ❖ Reduce heat to low and simmer partially covered for about 1 hour or until desired doneness
- ❖ Add the spinach, salt and black pepper and cook for about 4 minutes.
- ❖ Add the lemon juice and remove from heat.
- ❖ Serve hot.

45) VEGETARIAN STEW

Preparation Time: 20 minutes	Cooking Time: 35 minutes	Servings: 8

✓ 2 tablespoons of coconut oil ✓ 1 large sweet onion, chopped ✓ 1 medium parsnip, peeled and chopped ✓ 3 tablespoons of homemade tomato paste ✓ 2 large garlic cloves, minced ✓ ½ teaspoon ground cinnamon ✓ ½ teaspoon ground ginger ✓ 1 teaspoon of ground cumin ✓ ¼ teaspoon cayenne pepper	✓ 2 medium carrots, peeled and chopped ✓ 2 medium purple potatoes, peeled and cut into pieces ✓ 2 medium sweet potatoes, peeled and cut into pieces ✓ 4 cups of homemade vegetable broth ✓ 2 cups fresh cabbage, cut and chopped ✓ 2 tablespoons fresh lemon juice ✓ Sea salt and freshly ground black pepper, to taste

Directions: ❖ In a large soup pot, melt the coconut oil over medium-high heat and sauté the onion for about 5 minutes. ❖ Add the parsnips and sauté for about 3 minutes. ❖ Stir in the tomato paste, garlic and spices and sauté for about 2 minutes.	❖ Stir in the carrots, potatoes, sweet potatoes and broth and bring to a boil. ❖ Reduce the heat to medium-low and simmer covered for about 20 minutes. ❖ Stir in the cabbage, lemon juice, salt and black pepper and simmer for about 5 minutes. ❖ Serve hot.

46) QUINOA AND LENTIL STEW

Preparation Time: 15 minutes	Cooking Time: 30 minutes	Servings: 6

✓ 1 tablespoon of coconut oil ✓ 3 carrots, peeled and cut into pieces ✓ 3 celery stalks, chopped ✓ 1 yellow onion, chopped ✓ 4 garlic cloves, minced ✓ 4 cups of tomatoes, chopped ✓ 1 cup red lentils, rinsed and drained	✓ ½ cup dried quinoa, rinsed and drained ✓ 1½ teaspoons of ground cumin ✓ 1 teaspoon of red chili powder ✓ 5 cups of vegetable broth ✓ 2 cups fresh spinach, chopped ✓ Sea salt and freshly ground black pepper, to taste

Directions: ❖ In a large skillet, heat the oil over medium heat and sauté the celery, onion and carrot for about 4-5 minutes. ❖ Add the garlic and sauté for about 1 minute. ❖ Add the remaining ingredients except the spinach and bring to a boil.	❖ Reduce the heat to low and simmer covered for about 20 minutes. ❖ Add the spinach and simmer for about 3-4 minutes. ❖ Add the salt and black pepper and remove from heat. ❖ Serve hot.

47) BLACK BEAN CHILI

Preparation Time: 15 minutes		Servings: 6

✓ 2 tablespoons of olive oil ✓ 1 onion, chopped ✓ 1 small red bell pepper, seeded and chopped ✓ 1 small green bell pepper, seeded and chopped ✓ 4 garlic cloves, minced ✓ 1 teaspoon of ground cumin ✓ 1 teaspoon of cayenne pepper	✓ 1 tablespoon of red chili powder ✓ 1 medium sweet potato, peeled and cut into pieces ✓ 3 cups of tomatoes, finely chopped ✓ 4 cups of cooked, rinsed and drained black beans ✓ 2 cups of homemade vegetable broth ✓ Sea salt and freshly ground black pepper, to taste

Directions: ❖ In a large skillet, heat the oil over medium-high heat and sauté the onion and peppers for about 3-4 minutes. ❖ Add the garlic and spices and sauté for about 1 minute. ❖ Add the sweet potato and cook for about 4-5 minutes.	❖ Add the remaining ingredients and bring to a boil. ❖ Reduce heat to medium-low and simmer covered for about 1½-2 hours. ❖ Season with the salt and black pepper and remove from heat. ❖ Serve hot.

48) KIDNEY BEAN CURRY

Preparation Time: 15 minutes	Cooking Time: 25 minutes	Servings: 6

Ingredients:

- ¼ cup of extra virgin olive oil
- 1 medium onion, finely chopped
- 2 garlic cloves, minced
- 2 tablespoons fresh ginger, chopped
- 1 cup of homemade tomato puree
- 1 teaspoon of ground coriander
- 1 teaspoon of ground cumin
- ½ teaspoon ground turmeric

Ingredients:

- ¼ teaspoon cayenne pepper
- Sea salt and freshly ground black pepper, to taste
- 2 large plum tomatoes, finely chopped
- 3 cups of boiled red beans
- 2 cups of water
- ½ cup fresh parsley, chopped

Directions:

- ❖ In a large soup pot, heat the oil over medium heat and sauté the onion, garlic and ginger for about 4-5 minutes.
- ❖ Stir in the tomato puree and spices and cook for about 5 minutes.
- ❖ Add the tomatoes, beans and water and bring to a boil over high heat.

- ❖ Reduce heat to medium and simmer for about 10-15 minutes or until desired thickness.
- ❖ Serve hot and garnish with parsley.

49) GREEN BEANS IN CASSEROLE

Preparation Time: 20 minutes	Cooking Time: 20 minutes	Servings: 6

Ingredients:

For the onion slices:
- ½ cup yellow onion, very thinly sliced
- ¼ cup almond flour
- 1/8 teaspoon of garlic powder
- Sea salt and freshly ground black pepper, to taste

For the casserole:
- 1 pound fresh green beans, cut up
- 1 tablespoon of olive oil

Ingredients:

- 8 ounces fresh cremini mushrooms, sliced
- ½ cup yellow onion, thinly sliced
- 1/8 teaspoon of garlic powder
- Sea salt and freshly ground black pepper, to taste
- 1 teaspoon fresh thyme, chopped
- ½ cup homemade vegetable broth
- ½ cup of coconut cream

Directions:

- ❖ Preheat the oven to 350 degrees F.
- ❖ For the onion slices, place all ingredients in a bowl and toss to coat the onion well.
- ❖ Arrange the onion slices on a large baking sheet in a single layer and set aside.
- ❖ In a pot of boiling salted water, add the green beans and cook for about 5 minutes.
- ❖ Drain green beans and transfer to a bowl of ice water.
- ❖ Again, drain them well and transfer them back to a large bowl. Set them aside.
- ❖ In a large skillet, heat the oil over medium-high heat and sauté the mushrooms, onion, garlic powder, salt and black pepper for about 2-3 minutes.

- ❖ Stir in the thyme and broth and cook for about 3-5 minutes or until all the liquid is absorbed.
- ❖ Remove from heat and transfer the mushroom mixture to the bowl with the green beans.
- ❖ Add the coconut cream and stir to combine well.
- ❖ Transfer the mixture to a 10-inch casserole dish.
- ❖ Place the casserole dish and pan of onion slices in the oven.
- ❖ Bake for about 15-17 minutes.
- ❖ Remove the pan and sheet from the oven and let cool for about 5 minutes before serving.
- ❖ Top the casserole with the crispy onion slices evenly.
- ❖ Cut into 6 equal-sized portions and serve.

50) VEGETARIAN CAKE

Preparation Time: 20 minutes	Cooking Time: 20 minutes	Servings: 8

Ingredients:

For the gasket:
- ✓ 5 cups of water
- ✓ 1¼ cup yellow cornmeal

For archiving:
- ✓ 1 tablespoon of extra virgin olive oil
- ✓ 1 large onion, chopped
- ✓ 1 medium red bell pepper, seeded and chopped

Ingredients:

- ✓ 2 garlic cloves, minced
- ✓ 1 teaspoon dried oregano, crushed
- ✓ 2 teaspoons of chili powder
- ✓ 2 cups fresh tomatoes, chopped
- ✓ 2½ cups cooked pinto beans
- ✓ 2 cups of boiled corn kernels

Directions:

- ❖ Preheat oven to 375 degrees F. Lightly grease a shallow baking dish.
- ❖ In a skillet, add the water over medium-high heat and bring to a boil.
- ❖ Slowly add the cornmeal, stirring constantly.
- ❖ Reduce heat to low and cook covered for about 20 minutes, stirring occasionally.
- ❖ Meanwhile, prepare the filling. In a large skillet, heat the oil over medium heat and sauté the onion and bell bell pepper for about 3-4 minutes.
- ❖ Add garlic, oregano and spices and sauté for about 1 minute
- ❖ Add remaining ingredients and stir to combine.

- ❖ Reduce the heat to low and simmer for about 10-15 minutes, stirring occasionally.
- ❖ Remove from heat.
- ❖ Place half of the cooked cornmeal in the prepared baking dish evenly.
- ❖ Spoon the filling mixture over the cornmeal evenly.
- ❖ Place the remaining cornmeal on top of the filling mixture evenly.
- ❖ Bake for 45-50 minutes or until the top turns golden brown.
- ❖ Remove the cake from the oven and set aside for about 5 minutes before serving.

51) RICE AND LENTILS MEATLOAF

Preparation Time: 20 minutes	Cooking Time: 1 hours 10 minutes	Servings: 8

Ingredients:

- ✓ 1¾ cup plus 2 tablespoons of filtered water, divided
- ✓ ½ cup wild rice
- ✓ ½ cup of brown lentils
- ✓ Pinch of sea salt
- ✓ ½ teaspoon of sodium-free Italian seasoning
- ✓ 1 medium yellow onion, chopped
- ✓ 1 celery stalk, chopped
- ✓ 6 cremini mushrooms, chopped

Ingredients:

- ✓ 4 garlic cloves, minced
- ✓ ¾ cup rolled oats
- ✓ ½ cup pecans, finely chopped
- ✓ ¾ cup of homemade tomato sauce
- ✓ ½ teaspoon of red pepper flakes, crushed
- ✓ 1 teaspoon fresh rosemary, chopped
- ✓ 2 teaspoons fresh thyme, chopped

Directions:

- ❖ In a saucepan, add 1¾ cups water, the rice, lentils, salt and Italian seasoning and bring to a boil over medium-high heat.
- ❖ Reduce the heat to low and simmer covered for about 45 minutes.
- ❖ Remove from heat and set aside still covered for at least 10 minutes.
- ❖ Preheat the oven to 350 degrees F.
- ❖ Using the parchment paper, line a 9x5-inch baking dish.
- ❖ In a skillet, heat the remaining water over medium heat and sauté the onion, celery, mushrooms and garlic for about 4-5 minutes.
- ❖ Remove from heat and allow to cool slightly.

- ❖ In a large bowl, add the oats, pecans, tomato sauce and fresh herbs and stir until well combined.
- ❖ Combine the rice mixture and vegetable mixture with the oat mixture and mix well.
- ❖ In a blender, add the mixture and pulse until it forms a chunky mixture.
- ❖ Transfer the mixture to the prepared baking dish evenly.
- ❖ With a piece of foil, cover the pan and bake for about 40 minutes.
- ❖ Uncover and bake for about 15-20 minutes more or until the top turns golden brown.
- ❖ Remove from oven and set aside for about 5-10 minutes before slicing.
- ❖ Cut into desired size slices and serve.

52) ASPARAGUS RISOTTO

Preparation Time: 15 minutes	Cooking Time: 45 minutes	Servings: 4

✓ 15-20 fresh asparagus spears, trimmed and cut into 1½-inch pieces ✓ 2 tablespoons of olive oil ✓ 1 cup yellow onion, chopped ✓ 1 garlic clove, minced ✓ 1 cup of Arborio rice ✓ 1 tablespoon fresh lemon zest, finely grated	✓ 2 tablespoons fresh lemon juice ✓ 5½ cups hot vegetable broth ✓ 1 tablespoon fresh parsley, chopped ✓ ¼ cup nutritional yeast ✓ Sea salt and freshly ground black pepper, to taste

Directions:

❖ Boil water in a medium skillet then add asparagus and cook for about 3 minutes.
❖ Drain asparagus and rinse under cold running water.
❖ Drain well and set aside.
❖ In a large skillet, heat the oil over medium heat and sauté the onion for about 5 minutes.
❖ Add the garlic and sauté for about 1 minute.
❖ Add the rice and sauté for about 2 minutes.

❖ Add the lemon zest, lemon juice and ½ cup of the broth and cook for about 3 minutes or until all the liquid is absorbed, stirring gently.
❖ Add 1 cup broth and cook until all broth is absorbed.
❖ While stirring occasionally, repeat this process by adding ¾ cup of broth at a time until all the broth is absorbed. (This process will take about 20-30 minutes).
❖ Stir in the cooked asparagus and remaining ingredients and cook for about 4 minutes.
❖ Serve hot.

53) QUINOA AND CHICKPEA SALAD

Preparation Time: 15 minutes	Cooking Time: 45 minutes	Servings: 8

✓ 1¾ cup of homemade vegetable broth ✓ 1 cup quinoa, rinsed ✓ Sea salt, to taste ✓ 1½ cups of cooked chickpeas ✓ 1 medium green bell pepper, seeded and chopped ✓ 1 medium red bell pepper, seeded and chopped	✓ 2 cucumbers, chopped ✓ ½ cup shallots (green part only), chopped ✓ 1 tablespoon of olive oil ✓ 2 tablespoons fresh coriander leaves, chopped

Directions:

❖ In a skillet, add the broth and bring to a boil over high heat.
❖ Add the quinoa and salt and cook again until boiling.
❖ Reduce the heat to low and simmer covered for about 15-20 minutes or until all the liquid is absorbed.

❖ Remove from heat and set aside still covered for about 5-10 minutes.
❖ Uncover and stir the quinoa with a fork.
❖ In a large serving bowl, add the quinoa and remaining ingredients and toss gently to coat.
❖ Serve immediately.

54) MIXED VEGETABLE SOUP

✓ 1½ tablespoons of olive oil ✓ 4 medium carrots, peeled and chopped ✓ 1 medium onion, chopped ✓ 2 garlic cloves, minced ✓ 2 stalks of celery, chopped ✓ 2 cups fresh tomatoes, finely chopped	✓ 3 cups of small cauliflower florets ✓ 3 cups of small broccoli florets ✓ 3 cups frozen peas ✓ 8 cups of homemade vegetable broth ✓ 3 tablespoons fresh lemon juice ✓ Sea salt, to taste

Directions:

❖ In a large soup pot, heat the oil over medium heat and sauté the carrots, celery and onion for 6 minutes.
❖ Add the garlic and sauté for about 1 minute.
❖ Add the tomatoes and cook for about 2-3 minutes, crushing them with the back of a spoon.

❖ Add the vegetables and broth and bring to a boil over high heat.
❖ Reduce heat to a minimum.
❖ Cover the pot and simmer for about 30-35 minutes.
❖ Add the lemon juice and salt and remove from heat.
❖ Serve hot.

55) BEANS AND BARLEY SOUP

Preparation Time: 15 minutes	Cooking Time: 40 minutes	Servings: 4

- ✓ 1 tablespoon of olive oil
- ✓ 1 white onion, chopped
- ✓ 2 stalks of celery, chopped
- ✓ 1 large carrot, peeled and chopped
- ✓ 2 tablespoons fresh rosemary, chopped
- ✓ 2 garlic cloves, minced
- ✓ 4 cups fresh tomatoes, chopped

- ✓ 4 cups of homemade vegetable broth
- ✓ 1 cup pearl barley
- ✓ 2 cups of cooked white beans
- ✓ 2 tablespoons fresh lemon juice
- ✓ 4 tablespoons fresh parsley leaves, chopped

Directions:

- ❖ In a large soup pot, heat the oil over medium heat and sauté the onion, celery and carrot for about 4-5 minutes.
- ❖ Add the garlic and rosemary and sauté for about 1 minute.
- ❖ Add the tomatoes and cook for 3-4 minutes, crushing them with the back of a spoon.

- ❖ Add the barley and broth and bring to a boil.
- ❖ Reduce the heat to low and simmer covered for about 20-25 minutes.
- ❖ Add the beans and lemon juice and simmer for about 5 more minutes.
- ❖ Garnish with parsley and serve hot

56) TOFU AND BELL PEPPER STEW

Preparation Time: 15 minutes	Cooking Time: 15 minutes	Servings: 6

- ✓ 2 tablespoons of garlic
- ✓ 1 jalapeño bell pepper, seeded and chopped
- ✓ 1 (16-ounce) can of roasted, rinsed, drained and chopped red peppers
- ✓ 2 cups of homemade vegetable broth
- ✓ 2 cups of filtered water

- ✓ 1 medium green bell pepper, seeded and thinly sliced
- ✓ 1 medium red bell pepper, seeded and thinly sliced
- ✓ 1 (16-ounce) package of extra-firm tofu, drained and diced
- ✓ 1 (10-ounce) package of frozen spinach, thawed

Directions:

- ❖ Add the garlic, jalapeño bell pepper, and roasted red peppers to a food processor and pulse until smooth.
- ❖ In a large skillet, add the puree, broth and water and cook until boiling over medium-high heat.

- ❖ Add the peppers and tofu and stir to combine.
- ❖ Reduce the heat to medium and cook for about 5 minutes.
- ❖ Stir in the spinach and cook for about 5 minutes.
- ❖ Serve hot.

57) CHICKPEA STEW

Preparation Time: 15 minutes	Cooking Time: 30 minutes	Servings: 4

- ✓ 1 tablespoon of olive oil
- ✓ 1 medium onion, chopped
- ✓ 2 cups of carrots, peeled and chopped
- ✓ 2 garlic cloves, minced
- ✓ 1 teaspoon of red pepper flakes
- ✓ 2 large tomatoes, peeled, seeded and finely chopped

- ✓ 2 cups of homemade vegetable broth
- ✓ 2 cups of cooked chickpeas
- ✓ 2 cups fresh spinach, chopped
- ✓ 1 tablespoon fresh lemon juice
- ✓ Sea salt and freshly ground black pepper, to taste

Directions:

- ❖ In a large skillet, heat the oil over medium heat and sauté the onion and carrot for about 6 minutes.
- ❖ Add the garlic and red pepper flakes and sauté for about 1 minute.
- ❖ Add the tomatoes and cook for about 2-3 minutes.

- ❖ Add the broth and bring to a boil.
- ❖ Reduce the heat to low and simmer for about 10 minutes.
- ❖ Stir in the chickpeas and simmer for about 5 minutes.
- ❖ Add the spinach and simmer for another 3-4 minutes.
- ❖ Add the lemon juice and seasoning and remove from heat.
- ❖ Serve hot.

58) LENTILS WITH CABBAGE

Preparation Time: 15 minutes	Cooking Time: 20 minutes	Servings: 6

Ingredients:

- ✓ 1½ cups of red lentils
- ✓ 1½ cups homemade vegetable broth
- ✓ 1½ tablespoons of olive oil
- ✓ ½ cup onion, chopped
- ✓ 1 teaspoon fresh ginger, peeled and chopped

Ingredients:

- ✓ 2 garlic cloves, minced
- ✓ 1½ cups tomato, chopped
- ✓ 6 cups fresh cabbage, hard ends removed and chopped
- ✓ Sea salt and ground black pepper, to taste

❖ In a skillet, add the broth and lentils and bring to a boil over medium-high heat.
❖ Reduce the heat to low and simmer covered for about 20 minutes or until almost all the liquid is absorbed.
❖ Remove from heat and set aside still covered.

❖ Meanwhile, in a large skillet, heat the oil over medium heat and sauté the onion for about 5-6 minutes.
❖ Add the ginger and garlic and sauté for about 1 minute.
❖ Add the tomatoes and cabbage and cook for about 4-5 minutes.
❖ Add the lentils, salt and black pepper and remove from heat.
❖ Serve hot.

59) VEGETARIAN RATATOUILLE

Preparation Time: 20 minutes	Cooking Time: 45 minutes	Servings: 4

Ingredients:

- ✓ 6 ounces of homemade tomato paste
- ✓ 3 tablespoons of olive oil, divided
- ✓ ½ chopped onion
- ✓ 3 tablespoons minced garlic
- ✓ Sea salt and freshly ground black pepper, to taste
- ✓ ¾ cup filtered water
- ✓ 1 zucchini, cut into thin circles

Ingredients:

- ✓ 1 yellow pumpkin, cut in thin circles
- ✓ 1 eggplant, cut into thin circles
- ✓ 1 red bell pepper, with seeds and cut into thin circles
- ✓ 1 yellow bell pepper, with seeds and cut into thin circles
- ✓ 1 tablespoon fresh thyme leaves, chopped
- ✓ 1 tablespoon fresh lemon juice

❖ Preheat the oven to 375 degrees F.
❖ In a bowl, add the tomato paste, 1 tablespoon oil, onion, garlic, salt and black pepper and mix well.
❖ In the bottom of a 10x10-inch baking dish, spread tomato paste mixture evenly.

❖ Arrange the vegetable slices alternately, starting at the outer edge of the pan and working concentrically toward the center.
❖ Drizzle the vegetables with the remaining oil and lemon juice and sprinkle with salt and black pepper followed by the thyme.
❖ Arrange a piece of parchment paper over the vegetables.
❖ Bake for about 45 minutes.
❖ Serve hot.

60) BAKED BEANS

Preparation Time: 15 minutes	Cooking Time: 5 hours 5 minutes	Servings: 4

Ingredients:

- ✓ ¼ pound of dried lima beans, soaked overnight and drained
- ✓ ¼ pound of dried red beans, soaked overnight and drained
- ✓ 1¼ tablespoon of olive oil
- ✓ 1 small yellow onion, chopped
- ✓ 4 garlic cloves, minced
- ✓ 1 teaspoon dried thyme, crushed

Ingredients:

- ✓ ½ teaspoon of ground cumin
- ✓ ½ teaspoon of red pepper flakes, crushed
- ✓ ¼ teaspoon of smoked paprika
- ✓ 1 tablespoon fresh lemon juice
- ✓ 1 cup of homemade tomato sauce
- ✓ 1 cup homemade vegetable broth

❖ Add the beans to a large pot of boiling water and bring back to a boil.
❖ Reduce heat to a minimum.
❖ Cover the pan and bake for about 1 hour.
❖ Drain the beans well.
❖ Preheat the oven to 325 degrees F.

❖ In a large ovenproof skillet, heat the oil over medium heat and sauté the onion for about 4 minutes.
❖ Add the garlic, thyme and spices and sauté for about 1 minute.
❖ Stir in cooked beans and remaining ingredients and immediately remove from heat.
❖ Cover the pan and bake in the oven for about 1 hour.
❖ Serve hot.

61) BARLEY PILAF

Preparation Time: 20 minutes	Cooking Time: 1 hour 5 minutes	Servings: 4

✓ ½ cup of pearl barley	✓ ½ cup green bell bell pepper, seeded and chopped
✓ 1 cup of vegetable broth	✓ ½ cup red bell bell pepper, seeded and chopped
✓ 2 tablespoons vegetable oil, divided	✓ 2 tablespoons fresh cilantro, chopped
✓ 2 garlic cloves, minced	✓ 2 tablespoons fresh mint leaves, chopped
✓ ½ cup white onion, chopped	✓ 1 tablespoon of tamari
✓ ½ cup green olives, sliced	

❖ In a skillet, add the barley and broth over medium-high heat and cook until boiling.	❖ Remove from heat and set aside.
❖ Immediately, reduce the heat to low and simmer covered for about 45 minutes or until all the liquid has evaporated.	❖ In another skillet, heat the remaining oil over medium heat and sauté the onion for about 7 minutes.
❖ In a large skillet, heat 1 tablespoon oil over medium-high heat and sauté garlic for about 30 seconds.	❖ Add the olives and peppers and sauté for about 3 minutes.
❖ Stir in the cooked barley and cook for about 3 minutes.	❖ Stir in the remaining ingredients and cook for about 3 minutes.
	❖ Stir in the barley mixture and cook for about 3 minutes.
	❖ Serve hot.

62) KEBAB OF VEGETABLES AND SALMON

✓ 4 wooden skewers	✓ Pepper (.5 tsp.)
✓ Pepper (.25 tsp.)	✓ Salt (1 teaspoon)
✓ Salt (.5 tsp.)	✓ Olive oil (.25 c.)
✓ Chopped garlic cloves (1)	✓ Pumpkin seeds (.25 c.)
✓ Olive oil (1 tablespoon)	✓ Basil leaves (.5 c.)
✓ Sweet onion cut into quarters (.5)	✓ Chopped garlic clove (1)
✓ Sliced yellow bell pepper (1)	✓ Spinach (1 c.)
✓ Cherry Tomatoes (12)	✓ Lemon juice (1)
✓ Chopped zucchini (1)	
✓ Salmon (6 oz.)	
✓ For the plague sauce	

❖ Take out the skewers and thread the veggies and salmon through them the way you prefer.	❖ After 20 minutes, check to see if the fish is cooked and then set aside to cool.
❖ Place them in a baking dish and then brush on the pepper, garlic, salt and olive oil.	❖ Take out your blender and put in all the ingredients for the pesto sauce. Add more oil if needed.
❖ Turn on the oven and give it time to heat up to 400 degrees. Add the skewers to the oven and bake for a bit.	❖ Drizzle the pesto sauce over your salmon skewers before serving.

63) COCONUT CURRY WITH VEGETABLES

✓ Chopped coriander (3 tablespoons)	✓ Green beans (.25 lb.)
✓ Curry powder (2 teaspoons)	✓ Diced eggplant (.5 c.)
✓ Salt (1 teaspoon)	✓ Sliced yellow bell pepper (1)
✓ Water (.33 c.)	✓ Diced zucchini (2)
✓ Coconut milk (1 c.)	✓ Diced yellow onion (.5)
✓ Diced Tomato (1)	✓ Coconut oil (2 tablespoons)
✓ Firm tofu, sliced (8 ounces)	

❖ Take out a skillet and heat the coconut oil. When the oil is hot, add the beans, eggplant, peppers, zucchini, ginger and onion.	❖ After another 5 minutes, add the curry powder, salt, water and coconut milk. Let it simmer for a while.
❖ Cook these for five minutes, and then add the tomatoes and tofu. Stir to cook for a little longer.	❖ Ten minutes later, the dish is ready. Add the cilantro and enjoy!

64) SPAGHETTI SQUASH LOADED

Ingredients:

- ✓ Lemon peel (.5 tsp.)
- ✓ Torn basil leaves (1 c.)
- ✓ Salt (.5 tsp.)
- ✓ Oregano (.5 tsp.)
- ✓ Brown or green lentils, cooked (1 c.)

Ingredients:

- ✓ Diced Tomatoes (6)
- ✓ Chopped garlic cloves (1)
- ✓ Chopped Leek (1)
- ✓ Olive oil (1.5 tablespoons)
- ✓ Tagliata of spaghetti with pumpkin (1)

❖ After eight minutes, you can add the dried oregano and lentils, cooking for another 5 minutes.
❖ When the squash is ready, remove it from the oven and use a fork to separate the flesh.
❖ Add the lentil and vegetable mixture to this meat and combine.
❖ Add the olive oil, lemon zest and torn basil leaves before serving.

Directions:

❖ Turn on the oven and give it some time to heat up to 375 degrees. While it heats up, add a little oil to each spaghetti half and then place them face down on a baking sheet lined with parchment paper.
❖ Add the squash to the oven and let it cook until tender. After half an hour, the dish should be ready.
❖ While this is cooking, heat the rest of the oil in a skillet. Add the tomatoes, garlic, and leaks

65) SPICY PASTA

Preparation Time:

- ✓ Torn basil leaves (1 c.)
- ✓ Crushed pepper (1 teaspoon)
- ✓ Salt (1 teaspoon)
- ✓ Chili pepper diced (1)
- ✓ Sliced black olives (.5 c.)
- ✓ Diced zucchini (.5)
- ✓ Dried tomatoes cut into cubes (.5 c.)

- ✓ Diced cherry tomatoes (2 c.)
- ✓ Diced Carrot (1)
- ✓ diced celery stalks (1)
- ✓ Diced shallots (1)
- ✓ Chopped garlic cloves (1)
- ✓ Olive oil (3 tablespoons)
- ✓ Spelt dough (8 ounces)

❖ After eight minutes, add the zucchini, sun-dried tomatoes, cherry tomatoes, pepper, salt, chili and olives.
❖ When this is done, toss the pasta into the skillet and combine well. Move to a serving dish and top with a few basil leaves before serving.

Directions:

❖ Use the instructions on the package to cook the spelt noodles. Drain water and set aside.
❖ Add a little oil to a skillet before cooking the shallots, carrot, celery and garlic until soft.

66) STUFFED PEPPERS

- ✓ Peppers, cut tops (2)
- ✓ Crushed pepper (1 teaspoon)
- ✓ Salt (1 teaspoon)
- ✓ Chopped coriander (1 tablespoon)
- ✓ Lime Juice (.5)
- ✓ Chili powder (1 teaspoon)
- ✓ Cumin (1 teaspoon)

- ✓ Olive oil (2 tablespoons)
- ✓ Diced avocado (.5)
- ✓ Diced cucumber (1)
- ✓ Diced red bell pepper (1)
- ✓ Cooked green lentils (.5 c.)
- ✓ Cooked quinoa (1 c.)

❖ Pour this mixture over the lentil and quinoa mixture and stir. Use this mixture to stuff each bell pepper before serving.

Directions:

❖ Pull out a bowl and combine together the avocado, cucumber, diced bell bell pepper, lentil and quinoa.
❖ In another bowl, whisk together the salt, cilantro, lime juice, chili, cumin, pepper and olive oil.

67) BABA GANOUSH PASTA

Ingredients:

- ✓ Chopped parsley (.25 c.)
- ✓ Cayenne pepper (1 pinch)
- ✓ Salt (.5 tsp.)
- ✓ Vegetable stock (1 c.)
- ✓ Chopped chili pepper (1)
- ✓ Chopped garlic clove (1)
- ✓ Chopped Onion (1)

Ingredients:

- ✓ Diced red bell pepper (.5)
- ✓ Diced zucchini (1)
- ✓ Cubed eggplant (1)
- ✓ Olive oil (1 tablespoon)
- ✓ Spelt dough (6 ounces)

Directions:

- ❖ Follow the directions on the package to cook the farro pasta and then set it aside.
- ❖ Heat some oil in a skillet and when the oil is ready, add the chili, garlic, onion, bell bell pepper, zucchini and eggplant to the skillet.
- ❖ After 6 minutes of cooking, add the vegetable broth and cook for another 5 minutes or until hot.

- ❖ Take this out of the oven and give it a few minutes to cool before adding it to the blender. Blend until nice and smooth.
- ❖ Add the sauce to your skillet and season with a little pepper and salt. Add the cooked pasta and sprinkle with parsley before serving.

68) BOWL OF BROCCOLI WITH CHEESE

Ingredients:

- ✓ Crushed black pepper (.5 tsp.)
- ✓ Salt (.5 tsp.)
- ✓ Yeast nutrition (.24 c.)
- ✓ Lemon juice (1 tablespoon)

Ingredients:

- ✓ Cooked broccoli florets (4 c.)
- ✓ Cooked quinoa (1 c.)
- ✓ Olive oil (1 tablespoon)

Directions:

- ❖ To start this recipe, pull out a skillet and add the oil, broccoli, and cooked quinoa.

- ❖ Remove the dish from the heat and serve hot.
- ❖ After five minutes, this should be nice and hot, so add the pepper, salt, nutritional yeast and lemon juice.

69) GREEN BEAN AND LENTIL SALAD

Ingredients:

- ✓ Shallot (2 tablespoons)
- ✓ Apple Cider Vinegar (.25 c.)
- ✓ Sliced green beans (2 c.)
- ✓ Halved Cherry Tomatoes (1 c.)
- ✓ Cooked green lentils (2 c.)
- ✓ Pesto sauce

Ingredients:

- ✓ Salt (1 teaspoon)
- ✓ Olive oil (.25 c.)
- ✓ Chopped garlic clove (1)
- ✓ Pine nuts (2 tablespoons)
- ✓ Spinach (.5 c.)
- ✓ Basil leaves (.75 c.)

Directions:

- ❖ Take out the food processor and add all the ingredients for the pesto sauce to make it creamy and smooth.
- ❖ In another bowl, combine together the vinegar, green beans, tomatoes, lentils and scallions.

- ❖ Pour the pesto sauce over the mixture in the bowl, stir to coat, and then serve.

70) VEGETABLE SOUP

Ingredients:

- ✓ Spinach (1 c.)
- ✓ Basil (1 c.)
- ✓ Pepper (1 teaspoon)
- ✓ Salt (2 teaspoons)
- ✓ Oregano (1 tablespoon)
- ✓ Diced tomatoes (1 c.)
- ✓ Vegetable stock (1 c.)
- ✓ Kidney beans (.5 c.)

Ingredients:

- ✓ Chopped garlic clove (1)
- ✓ Shallot (1)
- ✓ Diced carrot (.5 c.)
- ✓ Diced zucchini (.5 c.)
- ✓ Diced pumpkin (.5 c.)
- ✓ Diced eggplant (.5 c.)
- ✓ Olive oil (1 tablespoon)

❖ Let these ingredients simmer together for another ten minutes, adding more spices if you like.
❖ Stir in the spinach and basil just before serving and enjoy.

Directions:

❖ Take out a stock pot and heat the olive oil inside. When the oil is hot, add the garlic, shallots, carrot, zucchini, squash, and eggplant to the pot.
❖ After five minutes of cooking, add the salt, oregano, diced tomatoes, broth, beans and pepper.

71) SOUTHWEST HAMBURGER

Ingredients:

- ✓ Sliced avocado (1)
- ✓ Lettuce Leaves, Bibb (2)
- ✓ Arugula (1 c.)
- ✓ Dijon mustard (1 tablespoon)
- ✓ Crushed walnuts (1 tablespoon)
- ✓ Nutritional yeast (1 tablespoon)
- ✓ Boiled tofu (4 ounces)
- ✓ Crushed black pepper (.5 tsp.)
- ✓ Cayenne pepper (.5 tsp.)

Ingredients:

- ✓ Ground Cumin (1 teaspoon)
- ✓ Salt (1 teaspoon)
- ✓ Diced Carrot (1)
- ✓ Diced green bell pepper (1 c.)
- ✓ Diced yellow onion (5.)
- ✓ Olive oil (1 tablespoon)

❖ Grate the tofu over the bowl and then add the Dijon mustard, walnuts and nutritional yeast. Mix everything together well and form into two burgers.
❖ Turn on the oven and let it heat to 400 degrees. Place the burgers on a paper-lined baking sheet and then add them to the oven.
❖ After half an hour, the burgers should be ready. Remove them from the oven and let them cool before topping with avocado and serving.

Directions:

❖ Heat some oil in a skillet. When the oil is hot, add the onion, pepper, cayenne, cumin, salt, carrot and bell bell pepper.
❖ After five minutes, the vegetables should be soft. Pour them into a bowl and let them cool.

72) ZUCCHINI ROLLS WITH RED SAUCE

Ingredients:

- ✓ Basil Leaves (15)
- ✓ Sliced zucchini (2)
- ✓ Water (.75 c.)
- ✓ Dried oregano (1 teaspoon)
- ✓ Salt (1 teaspoon)
- ✓ Diced red bell pepper (1)
- ✓ Diced Roma tomatoes (3)
- ✓ Chopped yellow onion (1)
- ✓ Olive oil (1 tablespoon)

Ingredients:

- ✓ Basil stuffing
- ✓ Chopped basil (1 handful)
- ✓ Nutmeg (.25 tsp.)
- ✓ Crushed pepper (.25 tsp.)
- ✓ Salt (.5 tsp.)
- ✓ Nutritional yeast (1 tablespoon)
- ✓ Water (3 tablespoons)
- ✓ Lemon juice (1)
- ✓ Soaked cashews (1 c.)

Directions:

- ❖ Get out a skillet and heat some oil in it. Add the oregano, salt, bell bell pepper, tomato and onion to make your red vegetable mixture.
- ❖ Cook for a few minutes to make the vegetables soft, and then add a little water. Let it simmer for a while.
- ❖ After ten minutes, remove the pan from the heat and give the vegetable mixture time to cool.
- ❖ Switch to a blender and blend until smooth.

- ❖ Now, work on the cashew filling. Clean the food processor and add all the ingredients until smooth. This can take some time, so be patient to do this.
- ❖ Place the zucchini ribbons on a plate in front of you and divide the filling between each one. Roll each ribbon tightly and then add it to an ovenproof dish with the red vegetable mixture on the bottom.
- ❖ Cover each of these rolls with the rest of the red vegetable mixture and add to the oven that is heated to 375 degrees.
- ❖ After 15 minutes, remove the pan from the oven and let the dish cool. Before serving, place the basil leaves on top and enjoy.

73) TACO WRAPS WITHOUT MEAT

Ingredients:

- ✓ Sliced avocado (.5)
- ✓ Romaine Leaves (4)
- ✓ Water (.25 c.)
- ✓ Salt (.5 tsp.)
- ✓ Cumin (.5 tsp.)
- ✓ Chilli powder (.5 tsp.)
- ✓ Smoked paprika (.5 tsp.)
- ✓ Chopped garlic clove (1)
- ✓ Tomato paste (1 tablespoon)
- ✓ Roasted walnuts (.5 c.)

Ingredients:

- ✓ Cooked brown lentils (1.5 c.)
- ✓ For the sauce
- ✓ Crushed pepper (.5 tsp.)
- ✓ Salt (.5 tsp.)
- ✓ Apple Cider Vinegar (1 tablespoon)
- ✓ Chopped coriander (3 tablespoons)
- ✓ Diced green bell pepper (.5 c.)
- ✓ Diced red bell pepper (.5 c.)
- ✓ Diced Mango (.5 c.)

Directions:

- ❖ Start with the sauce. Add all the ingredients into a bowl and stir to combine. Let it marinate for a bit while you work on your taco "meat".

- ❖ Take out the food processor and put together the water, salt, cumin, chili powder, paprika, garlic, tomato paste, walnuts, and lentils. You want this to still be a little crumbly when you're done.
- ❖ Place the walnut and lentil mixture in each romaine lettuce leaf, and then top with the salsa and avocado slices before serving.

74) SESAME AND QUINOA PILAF

Ingredients:

- ✓ Cooked green lentils (1 c.)
- ✓ Broth or water (1 c.)
- ✓ Quinoa (.5 c.)
- ✓ Chopped garlic clove (1)
- ✓ Diced green bell pepper (.5 c.)
- ✓ Diced celery stalk (1)
- ✓ Sliced shallot (1)
- ✓ Crushed pepper (2 teaspoons)
- ✓ Salt (2 teaspoons)
- ✓ Olive oil (2 tablespoons)
- ✓ Sliced carrots (2)

Ingredients:

- ✓ Green beans cut and sliced (1 c.)
- ✓ For the dressing
- ✓ Black sesame seeds (2 tablespoons)
- ✓ Rice vinegar (.25 c.)
- ✓ Tamari (.25 c.)
- ✓ Red pepper flakes (.5 tsp.)
- ✓ Lemon peel (1 teaspoon)
- ✓ Grated ginger (1 teaspoon)
- ✓ Toasted sesame oil (2 tablespoons)
- ✓ Avocado oil (.33 c.)

Directions:

- ❖ Add the carrots and green beans to some baking paper on a baking sheet. Sprinkle pepper, salt, and a tablespoon of olive oil on top.
- ❖ Add to the oven rack and bake until golden brown. This will take about five minutes.
- ❖ Once this is done, take a pot and add the garlic, bell bell pepper, celery, shallot and the rest of the oil.
- ❖ Cook the ingredients for five minutes before adding the quinoa and stirring to cook a little longer.

- ❖ Now, add the water or broth and bring to a boil. Let it simmer for a while until the liquid is gone.
- ❖ Now you can prepare the dressing. To do this, whisk together all the ingredients in a bowl to combine them.
- ❖ When it's time to assemble, mix together the quinoa and lentils. Season with a little pepper and salt and then add the carrot and bean mixture before pouring the dressing over the whole thing.

75) SMOKED SALMON WITH FRUIT SAUCE

Ingredients:

- ✓ Mixed vegetables (4 c.)
- ✓ Olive oil (1 tablespoon)
- ✓ Crushed pepper (.25 tsp.)
- ✓ Salt (.25 tsp.)
- ✓ Chilli powder (.5 tsp.)
- ✓ Garlic powder (1 teaspoon)
- ✓ Cayenne pepper (1 teaspoon)
- ✓ Salmon (8 ounces)

Ingredients:

- ✓ To make the sauce
- ✓ Halls
- ✓ Chopped coriander (1 tablespoon)
- ✓ Lime juice and zest (1)
- ✓ Diced pineapple (.5 c.)
- ✓ Diced Mango (.5 c.)
- ✓ Diced green bell pepper (.5)

Directions:

- ❖ Start this recipe by making the mango pineapple salsa. Add all ingredients to a bowl and stir to combine. Set aside for now.
- ❖ In another bowl, combine together the pepper, salt, chili powder, garlic powder and cayenne. Place this mixture on a flat plate to use at a moment's notice.

- ❖ Heat a skillet on the stove over medium heat. Brush olive oil all over the salmon fillet before adding the meat side to the spice mixture on the pan.
- ❖ Add the side of the meat to the pan and let it cook. After five minutes, turn the fish over and cook some more until the fish is done.
- ❖ Serve the fish with your chosen mixed vegetables and a little sauce on top.

76) ROCKET SALAD WITH SHRIMPS

Ingredients:

- ✓ Crushed black pepper (.5 tsp.)
- ✓ Salt (.5 tsp.)
- ✓ Chopped parsley (1 tablespoon)
- ✓ Chopped garlic clove (1)
- ✓ Olive oil (2 tablespoons)
- ✓ Lemon juice (.5)
- ✓ Shrimp (10)
- ✓ For the salad

Directions:

- ❖ Take out a bowl and add the pepper, parsley, salt, garlic, olive oil, lemon juice and shrimp. Place in the refrigerator to marinate for fifteen minutes or more.

Ingredients:

- ✓ Toasted pine nuts (2 tablespoons)
- ✓ Salt (1 teaspoon)
- ✓ Olive oil (2 tablespoons)
- ✓ Lemon juice (.5)
- ✓ Apple Cider Vinegar (2 tablespoons)
- ✓ Cherry Tomatoes Halved (10)
- ✓ Arugula (4 c.)

- ❖ When you are ready, take out a frying pan and heat it up. Add the prepared shrimp inside and cook a little on each side until the shrimp are all cooked through.
- ❖ Now it's time to prepare the salad. Get out a large salad bowl and combine all the salad ingredients together.
- ❖ Add the shrimp on top of the salad and serve warm.

77) EASY PIZZA

Ingredients:

- ✓ Lemon juice (1 teaspoon)
- ✓ Salt (1 teaspoon)
- ✓ Nutritional yeast (2 tablespoons)
- ✓ Olive oil (2 tablespoons)
- ✓ Arugula (1 c.)
- ✓ Sliced Tomato (1)
- ✓ Sliced avocado (1)

  For the pasta
- ✓ Dried basil (1 teaspoon)

Directions:

- ❖ Take out a blender and puree the sunflower seeds a couple of times. Then add them to a large bowl along with the basil, oregano, salt, pepper, olive oil, garlic and flaxseed meal.
- ❖ Knead this mixture until a nice dough forms. You can add more water if needed.
- ❖ Roll out the dough into a pizza shape. Place some baking paper on your baking sheet and place the dough on top.

Ingredients:

- ✓ Dried oregano (1 teaspoon)
- ✓ Pepper (1 teaspoon)
- ✓ Salt (1 teaspoon)
- ✓ Olive oil (4 tablespoons)
- ✓ Chopped garlic clove (1)
- ✓ Ground linseed (.33 c.)
- ✓ Sunflower seeds, soaked (1.25 c.)

- ❖ Heat your oven to the lowest temperature it will allow and then place the pan inside to dehydrate the dough. Give this about 12 hours to finish.
- ❖ When the dough is ready, you can put the tomato slices and avocado on top of the crust.
- ❖ Cough up the arugula in a small bowl with the lemon juice, salt, nutritional yeast and olive oil. Place this on top of the pizza and serve immediately.

78) SPELT BREAD

Ingredients:

- ✓ 3/4 - 1 cup of alkaline water
- ✓ ½ cup unsweetened hemp milk
- ✓ 3 tablespoons of avocado oil

Directions:

- ❖ Preheat oven to 375 degrees F. Meanwhile, combine all dry contents in a bowl.
- ❖ Add ¾ cup water, the hemp milk and avocado oil until fully blended to create a smooth batter.
- ❖ In case the batter seems rather stiff, add a few tablespoons of alkaline water until the dough is soft. And if it's too wet, add a few more tablespoons of spelt flour, stirring after each spoonful until the dough holds together well.
- ❖ Cover the work surface with about ½ cup of spelt flour. Then knead the dough on the floured surface and roll it to coat it with flour.
- ❖ Knead the dough for another 2 to 3 minutes, and add a little more spelt with each addition until you have a unified ball that can come back when prodded.

Ingredients:

- ✓ 1 tablespoon of agave nectar
- ✓ 1 ½ teaspoon of fine sea salt
- ✓ 4 cups of spelt flour + ½ cup more for kneading

- ❖ At this point, take a parchment paper and line a standard baking sheet across its width. Get some avocado oil and grease the ends of the baking sheet as well.
- ❖ Turn the dough into the prepared pan and pat it to distribute it well in the pan. Score the top of the loaf using a sharp knife, lengthwise.
- ❖ Finally, bake the bread until cooked through, or for about 45 minutes.
- ❖ Remove from the oven and insert a toothpick into the center of the bread. If the toothpick or a thin, sharp knife doesn't come out clean, bake for another 5 to 10 minutes.
- ❖ Let the loaf of bread cool completely in the baking dish and then cut it into slices. Serve it with some of the soup and top it with the avocado. Also sprinkle with smoked paprika and lemon if you like.

79) GREEN GODDESS BOWL WITH AVOCADO DRESSING

Preparation Time:	Cooking Time:	Servings: 4

For the salad:
- ✓ 2 tablespoons of hemp seeds
- ✓ 1/3 cup cherry tomatoes, halved
- ✓ ½ cup of kelp noodles, soaked and drained
- ✓ ½ zucchini
- ✓ 3 cups of cabbage, chopped
- ✓ Avocado dressing:
- ✓ A pinch of cayenne pepper
- ✓ 1 tablespoon of extra virgin olive oil
- ✓ ¼ teaspoon of sea salt
- ✓ 1 cup of filtered water

- ✓ 2 limes, freshly squeezed
- ✓ 1 tablespoon of dried sage
- ✓ 1 avocado
- ✓ Tahini Lemon Dressing:
- ✓ 1 tablespoon of extra virgin olive oil
- ✓ ¾ teaspoon of sea salt
- ✓ 1 fennel bulb
- ✓ ½ fresh squeezed lemon
- ✓ ½ cup of filtered water
- ✓ ¼ cup tahini, sesame butter
- ✓ Cayenne pepper to taste

Directions:

- ❖ First make zucchini noodles using a spiralizer.
- ❖ Then lightly steam the kale for about 4 minutes and set aside.
- ❖ Combine the kelp noodles with the zucchini noodles and toss together with the avocado and cumin dressing.

- ❖ Now add the cherry tomatoes and mix well. Plate the steamed broccoli and cabbage and top with the tahini dressing.
- ❖ Serve the cabbage with the tomatoes and noodles sprinkled with hemp seeds.

80) ASIAN SESAME DRESSING AND NOODLES

		Servings: 2

- ✓ 1 bag of Kelp Noodles or 1 zucchini to make the noodles
- ✓ 1 tablespoon raw sesame seeds, for garnish
- ✓ 1 shallot, chopped
- ✓ Parsnip, optional
- ✓ Sliced red bell pepper, optional

For the dressing:
- ✓ 1 fennel bulb, chopped
- ✓ ½ teaspoon lemon, freshly squeezed
- ✓ ½ teaspoon of agave sugar
- ✓ 2 tablespoons of tahini, sesame butter

- ❖ Pour the sesame dressing over the scallions and noodles, and mix well. Top with the sesame, if you like, and enjoy.

Directions:

- ❖ With a vegetable peeler or spiralizer, cut strips the size of a noodle or use 1 bag of kelp noodles.
- ❖ Mix all the ingredients for the dressing in a bowl, and mix well with a spoon. If using kelp noodles, place them in hot water for about 10 minutes to soften them.

81) INSTANT ALKALINE SUSHI ROLL UP

		Servings: 2

Ingredients:

For Dip/Hummus
- ✓ 1 fennel bulb
- ✓ A drop of olive oil
- ✓ 1 pinch of dried sage
- ✓ 1 tablespoon of tahini
- ✓ A handful of walnuts
- ✓ 100 g of chickpeas/garbanzos from a can, drained
- ✓ Pinch of Himalayan salt
- ✓ Juice of 1/2 lemon

Ingredients:

For Roll-Ups
- ✓ 1 bell pepper cut into matchsticks
- ✓ 1 small bunch of culantro
- ✓ 1 avocado, peeled and sliced
- ✓ 1 cucumber, cut into matchsticks
- ✓ 1 parsnip, cut into matchsticks
- ✓ 2 medium courgettes/courts

Directions:

- ❖ In a blender or food processor, blend all the ingredients for the hummus. Add a little lemon and olive oil in equal amounts until you get the desired consistency.
- ❖ To make the alkaline rolls, first cut the zucchini or squash into long, thin strips with a vegetable peeler.

- ❖ Lay out individual zucchini strips and spread a generous amount of almond hummus on the zucchini strip.
- ❖ Now add small amounts of avocado, strainer, and vegetable matches.
- ❖ Top with a few sesame seeds and then serve.

82) SPAGHETTI STUFFED WITH QUINOA

		Servings: 2

- ✓ 1 teaspoon chopped ginger
- ✓ 2 teaspoons of dried thyme
- ✓ 1 and 1/2 cup cooked quinoa
- ✓ 1/4 cup chopped walnuts
- ✓ 2 spring onions, white part, sliced
- ✓ 1 orange or red bell pepper

- ✓ 1 medium shallot
- ✓ 1 cup steamed green peas
- ✓ 2 tablespoons of coconut oil
- ✓ 1 large pumpkin or two smaller pumpkins
- ✓ Sea salt and cayenne pepper to taste

Directions:

- ❖ Preheat the oven to 400 degrees F.
- ❖ Then clean the pumpkins, cut them in half and then discard the seeds. Bake the squash for about 40 minutes or until tender.
- ❖ Meanwhile, in a skillet, heat a tablespoon of coconut oil and cook the bell bell pepper and chopped shallots until soft.

- ❖ Then add the cooked quinoa, green peas, spices and nuts and cook until heated through. Season the mixture with salt and pepper.
- ❖ At this point, divide the mixture among the squash and bake until cooked through, or for about 5-8 minutes.
- ❖ Remove from heat and serve the stuffed noodles with fresh vegetables such as cabbage.

83) SPELT PASTA WITH SPICY EGGPLANT SAUCE

		Servings: 2

- ✓ A little cold-pressed extra virgin olive oil
- ✓ 1 pinch of cayenne pepper
- ✓ 1/2 teaspoon of organic sea salt
- ✓ 1 handful of fresh basil
- ✓ 1 cup of vegetable broth
- ✓ 1 small hot pepper

- ✓ 1 fennel bulb
- ✓ 1 medium-sized onion
- ✓ 1 fresh red bell pepper
- ✓ 1 fresh eggplant
- ✓ 1 cup of spelt pasta

Directions:

- ❖ Cook spelt pasta according to package instructions.
- ❖ Meanwhile, cut the bell bell pepper and eggplant into cubes and then chop the basil, fennel bulb, onion and chili into small pieces.
- ❖ In a skillet, heat some olive oil and then sauté the fennel bulb and onions for a few minutes.
- ❖ Add the pepper cubes and eggplant along with the chili and cook for another 2 to 3 minutes.

- ❖ At this point dissolve the vegetable stock in 1 cup of alkaline water then add the mixture to the pan.
- ❖ Simmer the contents, stirring a few times, for about 10 minutes over low heat.
- ❖ Add the basil and season with a little pepper and salt. Spread the sauce over the farro pasta and enjoy!

84) SESAME CABBAGE WITH CHICKPEAS

		Servings: 2

✓ 1 tablespoon of sesame oil	✓ 1 bunch of green onions, thinly sliced
✓ 1 tablespoon of sesame seeds	✓ 2 tablespoons of olive oil
✓ 2 tablespoons of lemon juice	✓ Salt to taste
✓ 15 ounces of chickpea beans	✓ 1 bunch of cabbage
✓ 1 fennel bulb, chopped	

Directions:

❖ Start by cutting up the cabbage. Tear the leaves off the stem, roll them up and cut them into small pieces.

❖ Add some olive oil to a skillet and then sauté the green onions and fennel over low heat for about 1 minute.

❖ Add the beans and sauté for another 4 to 5 minutes. Add the cabbage, lemon juice and season with a little salt.

❖ Cook until the cabbage has reduced in size. Serve the cabbage, drizzle with a little sesame oil and a few sesame seeds.

85) ALKALINE VEGAN MEATLOAF

		Servings: 1 loaf of bread

✓ 1 cup of prepared wild rice	✓ 1 teaspoon of thyme
✓ 1/2 cup homemade tomato sauce, divided	✓ 1 teaspoon of sage
✓ 1/2 cup chopped yellow or white onion, divided	✓ 1 tablespoon of sea salt
✓ 1/2 cup chopped green bell pepper, split	✓ 1 tablespoon of onion powder
✓ 1 shallot, coarsely chopped	✓ 1 cup of chickpea or spelt flour
✓ 2 cups mixed mushrooms, coarsely chopped	✓ 1.5 cups of breadcrumbs (spelt flour)
✓ 1/4 teaspoon of cloves	✓ 2 cups of cooked chickpeas
✓ 1/2 teaspoon of ginger	✓ Cayenne to taste
✓ 1/2 teaspoon of tarragon	

Directions:

❖ Clean and dry the wild rice as required. Also prepare the chickpeas and set aside.

❖ Mix the chickpea flour or spelt flour with the bread crumbs and set the mixture aside.

❖ Chop green peppers and onions and place half of each on the side.

❖ Now chop the scallions and mushrooms and add them to a food processor; along with the chickpeas, half of the onion, half of the green peppers and the spices.

❖ Pulse the mixture until it is fully incorporated. Then add 2 tablespoons of tomato sauce and the wild rice, and continue to blend until you have a coarse paste.

❖ Move the mixture to a bowl large enough to accommodate the remaining flour, bread crumbs, onion and green pepper. Stir until everything is combined.

❖ At this point, place the mixture in a greased baking dish and cover with the remaining tomato sauce.

❖ Bake in a preheated 350 degree F oven for about 60-70 minutes, keeping an eye on the top so it doesn't burn.

❖ Then remove from oven and let cool for about 30 minutes. Serve with some sauce and vegetables and enjoy.

86) ALKALINE PIZZA CRUST

		Servings: 4

✓ 1 cup of spring water	✓ Cherry Tomatoes
✓ 2 teaspoons of grape oil	✓ Onions
✓ 2 teaspoons of agave	For Pizza Sauce
✓ 1 teaspoon of sea salt	✓ 1/2 teaspoon of oregano
✓ 1 teaspoon of onion powder	✓ 1/2 teaspoon of sea salt
✓ 1 1/2 cups of spelt flour	✓ 1/2 teaspoon of onion powder
✓ 2 teaspoons of sesame seeds	✓ 2 tablespoons chopped onion
✓ Gaskets (optional)	✓ 1 avocado
✓ 1 teaspoon of oregano	✓ Pinch of basil

❖ First, preheat the oven to 400 degrees F.

❖ In a medium sized bowl, mix all ingredients with ½ cup water.

❖ Add more water in small amounts until the dough rolls into a ball, or add more flour if the dough seems fluid.

❖ Coat a baking sheet with oil and add a little flour to your hands.

❖ Now roll out the thick dough in the baking dish and brush the top with extra grapeseed oil.

❖ Using a fork, poke a few holes in the dough and bake it in the preheated oven for about 10-15 minutes.

❖ Meanwhile, start making the avocado pizza sauce. *** (recipe included)

❖

❖ Once the crust is cooked, add the pizza sauce and any alkali friendly toppings you want, such as cherry tomatoes, onions, etc.

❖ Bake until cooked through, or for another 15-20 minutes.

❖ For Pizza Sauce

❖ To make the avocado pizza sauce, first cut the avocado in the middle, discard the core and then scrape the avocado flesh in a food processor

❖ Add all other sauce ingredients and process until smooth or about 3 minutes.

❖ Scrape the inside of the food processor once necessary.

87) ALKALINE VEGAN ELECTRIC CHOPS

		Servings: 1

✓ Grape oil	✓ 1/4 teaspoon of cayenne powder
✓ 1/2 teaspoon of cayenne	✓ 1/2 teaspoon ground ginger
✓ 1 teaspoon of onion powder	✓ 2 teaspoons of onion powder
✓ 1 teaspoon of sea salt	✓ 2 teaspoons of smoked sea salt/sea salt
✓ 1/4 cup of spring water	✓ 1/4 cup white onions, chopped
✓ 2 Portobello mushrooms	✓ 1/4 cup of date sugar
✓ 1/2 cup alkaline barbecue sauce	✓ 2 tablespoons of agave
✓ For the alkaline electric barbecue sauce	✓ 6 cherry tomatoes
✓ Servings: about 8-10 ounces	
✓ 1/8 teaspoon of cloves	

❖ First, remove the gills from the bottom of the individual mushroom caps and then slice the Portobello about ½ inch apart. ❖ Place sauce ingredients in a blender and puree until smooth. ❖ Add the sliced mushrooms to a container along with the water, a large amount of barbeque sauce and seasoning. ❖ Cover the mixture and keep it chilled for about 6-8 hours. Be sure to turn it at regular 2 hour intervals.	❖ Take a skewer and push about 3 Portobello mushrooms around the center, then take another skewer and repeat. If any slices of mushroom break off, reserve them as ribs. ❖ Brush a griddle with grapeseed oil and then cook the ribs over medium heat for about 12-15 minutes. Remember to flip them regularly, after every 3 minutes. ❖ Brush with more sauce after a few tosses and serve with your favorite alkaline dish.

88) WALNUT MEAT

		Servings: 6

✓ 1/2 cup fresh thyme, chopped	✓ 1 small red onion, chopped
✓ 1/2 teaspoon of sea salt	✓ 1 1/2 cups red bell pepper, chopped
✓ 1 pinch of dried basil	✓ 4 cups of soaked walnuts

❖ First, soak the nuts in spring water for at least 4 hours, or preferably overnight. ❖ Add the soaked walnuts to the food processor along with the bell bell pepper and onions. ❖ Add the salt and thyme and process on high speed until you reach your preferred consistency, either smooth or chunky.	❖ Transfer the mixture to a bowl using a rubber spatula and dehydrate to make a walnut crumble or meatballs. ❖ You can also add the contents to an airtight container and store it in the refrigerator for up to 1 week.

89) ELECTRIC ALKALINE STEAK WITH MUSHROOMS AND CHEESE

		Servings: 4

Mushroom mix:	For the cheese:
✓ 1 teaspoon of savory	✓ 1/2 teaspoon of basil
✓ 1 teaspoon of thyme	✓ 1/2 teaspoon of sea salt
✓ 1 teaspoon of oregano	✓ 1/2 teaspoon of oregano
✓ 1 teaspoon of smoked sea salt	✓ 1/2 teaspoon of cayenne powder
✓ 1 tablespoon of onion powder	✓ 1 1/2 teaspoon of onion powder
✓ 1 tablespoon of grape oil	✓ 1 1/2 teaspoon of hemp seeds
✓ 1/2 cup of alkaline electric garlic sauce	✓ 1/3 - 1/2 cup of spring water
✓ 1 cup of red peppers	✓ 3/4 cup Brazil nuts, soaked
✓ 1 cup green peppers	
✓ 1 cup onions, sliced	
✓ 4 mushroom caps	

Directions: ❖ First, slice the mushrooms to about 1/8 inch thickness. Then, in a bowl, whisk the sauce together with the seasonings to make a marinade. ❖ Dip the sliced portabella mushrooms into the marinade and let them sit for about 30 minutes. Stir after about 15 minutes.	❖ To make the "cheese", blend all ingredients in a blender until fully incorporated. ❖ Meanwhile, add the grapeseed oil to a skillet over medium heat and sauté the peppers and onions for about 3-5 minutes. ❖ Then add the marinated portabellas and sauté for another 5 minutes. Serve the cheese steak with a flatbread and enjoy.

90) ALKALINE ELECTRIC CHICKPEA TOFU

Preparation Time:	Cooking Time:	Servings: 2

Ingredients:

- ✓ 1 teaspoon of culantro
- ✓ 1 teaspoon of sea salt

Ingredients:

- ✓ 1 cup of chickpea flour
- ✓ 2 cups of spring water

Directions:

- ❖ First, line a baking sheet with baking paper.
- ❖ Then in a saucepan, continuously whisk all of the above ingredients together over medium heat until oatmeal-like, or about 3-5 minutes.
- ❖ Pour batter into a baking dish and flatten with a spatula.

- ❖ Let it cool until firm, or for about 30 minutes. You can keep it in the fridge to speed up the process.
- ❖ Once it's firm enough, place the tofu on a cutting board and cut it into cubes.
- ❖ Serve as is or bake or saute for a few more minutes. Season as you like and serve.

91) FOO YUNG ALKALINE ELECTRIC EGG

		Servings: 6

Ingredients:

- ✓ Grape oil
- ✓ 1 cup of spring water
- ✓ 1/8 teaspoon of ginger powder
- ✓ 1/2 teaspoon of cayenne powder
- ✓ 1 teaspoon of oregano
- ✓ 1 teaspoon of sea salt
- ✓ 1 teaspoon of onion powder
- ✓ 1 teaspoon of basil

Ingredients:

- ✓ 3/4 cup of chickpea flour
- ✓ 1/2 cup red and white onion, chopped
- ✓ 1/2 cup green onions, chopped
- ✓ 1/2 cup red and green peppers, chopped
- ✓ 1 cup butternut squash, chopped
- ✓ 2 cups mushrooms, sliced
- ✓ 3 cups of prepared spaghetti

Directions:

- ❖ Start by whisking the seasonings, chickpea flour and spring water in a bowl.
- ❖ Then add the vegetables and prepared noodles. Combine with your hands until everything is incorporated.
- ❖ Using the grapeseed oil, coat a large skillet well over high heat and then add ½ cup of the squash and vegetable mixture.

- ❖ Cut the mixture into patties and cook them in the hot skillet until golden brown, or about 3 to 4 minutes on each side. Add more oil if needed.
- ❖ Serve the egg foo yung with fried wild rice and alkaline friendly sauce and enjoy.

92) ALKALINE PASTA SALAD

	Cooking Time:	Servings: 4

Ingredients:

- ✓ 1/4 cup black olives
- ✓ 1/2 cup cherry tomatoes, cut in half
- ✓ 1/2 cup onions, diced
- ✓ 1 cup zucchini/summer squash, sliced

Ingredients:

- ✓ 1 cup red/yellow/green peppers, diced
- ✓ 4 cups of cooked spelt pasta
- ✓ 3/4 to 1 cup of alkaline electric "garlic" sauce

Directions:

- ❖ In a large bowl, mix all ingredients until well incorporated.

- ❖ Serve and enjoy.

93) MUSHROOMS "CHICKEN TENDERS

		Servings: 6

Ingredients:

- ✓ Grape oil
- ✓ 1 teaspoon of ground cloves
- ✓ 1 teaspoon of cayenne powder
- ✓ 2 teaspoons of ginger powder
- ✓ 2 teaspoons of onion powder
- ✓ 2 teaspoons of sage
- ✓ 2 teaspoons of sea salt

Ingredients:

- ✓ 2 teaspoons of basil
- ✓ 2 teaspoons of oregano
- ✓ 1 1/2 cup of spelt flour
- ✓ 1 1/2 cups of spring water
- ✓ 2-6 portabella, oyster or white mushrooms

Directions:

- ❖ First, slice the caps off the portabella, oyster or white mushrooms about 1/2 inch apart and add them to a large bowl. You can also slice the mushroom stems to make nuggets.
- ❖ Add some grapeseed oil, water and half of the individual seasonings to the bowl and let the mixture marinate for about 1 hour.
- ❖ In a separate bowl, mix the rest of the seasonings with the spelt flour and then batter the mushrooms.
- ❖ If baking, preheat the oven to 400 degrees F.

- ❖ Meanwhile, grease a baking sheet with grapeseed oil and then place the mushrooms on the baking sheet.
- ❖ Cook each side until crispy, turning once, or about 15 minutes per side. Serve.
- ❖ If using a stove, heat a skillet over medium-high heat. Then add about 3 tablespoons of grapeseed oil to the skillet.
- ❖ Cook the mushrooms until crispy, or for about 3 to 4 minutes per side. Be careful not to burst the oil due to high heat or liquid from the mushrooms. Enjoy!

94) PIZZA MARGARITA

		Servings: 6

Ingredients:

Crust:
- ✓ 1 1/2 cups of spelt flour
- ✓ 1 cup of spring water
- ✓ 1/2 teaspoon of onion powder
- ✓ 1/2 teaspoon of oregano
- ✓ 1/2 teaspoon of sea salt
- ✓ 1/2 teaspoon of basil

Cheese:
- ✓ 1/4 teaspoon of sea salt
- ✓ 1/2 teaspoon of basil
- ✓ 1/2 teaspoon of oregano

Ingredients:

- ✓ 1/2 teaspoon of onion powder
- ✓ 1 teaspoon of lime juice
- ✓ 1/4 cup hemp/nut milk
- ✓ 1/2 cup of spring water
- ✓ 1 cup of Brazil nuts, soaked for more than 2 hours

Gaskets:
- ✓ Alkaline Electric Tomato Sauce
- ✓ Red onion, sliced
- ✓ Plum tomatoes, sliced

Directions:

- ❖ In a medium bowl, combine all the seasonings with the spelt flour and then add half a cup of water.
- ❖ Add more water in small amounts until the dough can become a ball, or add more spelt flour if you find the dough wet.
- ❖ Roll the dough on a floured surface, in one direction as you turn it and turn it over after a couple of rolls. Keep adding spelt flour after turning to keep the dough from getting too sticky.
- ❖ Place the dough in a baking dish gently coated with oil, poking holes with a fork, and now bake in a preheated 350 degree oven for about 10-15 minutes.

- ❖ Meanwhile, add all the ingredients for the cheese to a blender, and process until smooth, or about 1 to 2 minutes.
- ❖ As soon as the crust is cooked, top it with the cheese, alkaline electric sauce and your favorite toppings. Add more cheese and sauce if you like.
- ❖ Bake the contents on the bottom of the grill at 425 degrees F for another 10-15 minutes. Enjoy!!!

95) ALKALINE ELECTRIC VEGETARIAN LASAGNA

		Servings: 6

Ingredients:

Pasta
- ✓ Spelt lasagna sheets
- ✓ Tomato sauce
- ✓ 1/2 teaspoon of cayenne powder
- ✓ 2 teaspoons of sea salt
- ✓ 2 teaspoons of oregano
- ✓ 2 teaspoons of basil
- ✓ 1 tablespoon of onion powder
- ✓ 1 tablespoon of agave
- ✓ 12 plumcake tomatoes
- ✓ "Meat Alternative
- ✓ 1 teaspoon of fennel powder
- ✓ 2 teaspoons of basil
- ✓ 2 teaspoons of oregano
- ✓ 1 tablespoon of sea salt
- ✓ 2 tablespoons of onion powder

Ingredients:

- ✓ 1/2 cup of tomato sauce
- ✓ 1 cup diced green, yellow, and red peppers
- ✓ 1 cup onions, chopped
- ✓ 1 cup of cooked chickpeas (garbanzo beans)
- ✓ 2 cups of cooked spelt berries/kernels
- ✓ Brazil nut cheese
- ✓ 1 teaspoon of basil
- ✓ 1 teaspoon of oregano
- ✓ 1 teaspoon of sea salt
- ✓ 1 tablespoon of onion powder
- ✓ 1 tablespoon of hemp seeds
- ✓ 1 cup of spring water
- ✓ 2 cups of soaked Brazil nuts
- ✓ Extra
- ✓ White mushrooms
- ✓ Grape oil
- ✓ Zucchini

Directions:

- ❖ Add the ingredients for the tomato sauce to a blender and then process until well combined.
- ❖ Add the grapeseed oil to a saucepan with the tomato sauce and heat the sauce over medium heat. Lower the heat and simmer until the sauce has thickened, or for 2 hours, stirring regularly.
- ❖ In a food processor, combine the ingredients for the "meat" which are the chickpea beans, farro and seasonings until well incorporated.
- ❖ Lightly coat a skillet with oil and heat it over medium heat. Sauté the peppers and onions for about 5 minutes.
- ❖ Now add the chickpea and farro mixture from the food processor, and a little grapeseed oil to the pan and cook the mixture until it begins to brown, or for 10-12 minutes.
- ❖ In a blender, add the remaining cheese ingredients along with 1 cup of water and process until well blended. If you find it too thick, add ¼ cup of spring water at a time until you get the consistency you want.

- ❖ Reserve one cup of tomato sauce, and then pour the rest of the sauce into the chickpea and farro mixture. Combine well.
- ❖ Slice the zucchini and mushrooms lengthwise. You can also make lasagna with zucchini instead of spelt pasta, if you like.
- ❖ At this point, start preparing the lasagna. Lightly coat the bottom of the dish with the reserved tomato sauce to make sure it doesn't stick.
- ❖ Then you roll out the spelt dough, sliced zucchini, chickpea and spelt mixture, alkaline cheese, white mushrooms and spelt dough again.
- ❖ Repeat this arrangement until you have 4 layers of dough. Then, top the last layer with the chickpea and farro mixture and the cheese.
- ❖ Pour the rest of the tomato sauce around the lasagna layers and sprinkle with a little dried basil if you like.
- ❖ Bake the whole thing at 350 degrees F for about 35-45 minutes.
- ❖ Then let the lasagna cool for about 15 minutes and then serve.

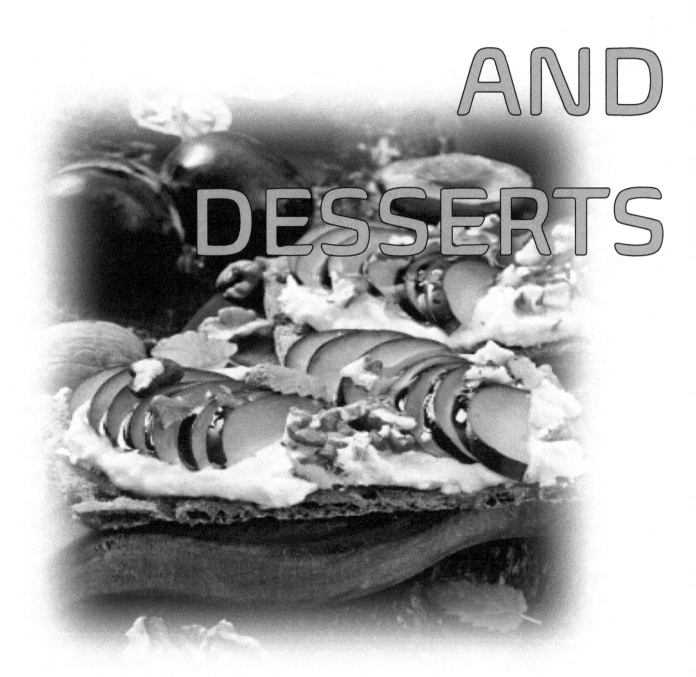

Chapter 4. SNACK AND DESSERTS

96) STRAWBERRY SORBET

Preparation Time: 4 hours		Servings: 4
✓ 2 cups of Strawberries*. ✓ 1 1/2 teaspoons of spelt flour		✓ 1/2 cup of sugar Date ✓ 2 cups of Spring Water
❖ Add the sugar Date, water and flour Spelt in a saucepan and simmer for about ten minutes. The mixture should look like syrup. ❖ Remove the meat from the cap and let it rest. ❖ After cooling, add Strawberry puree and gently mix. ❖ Place this mixture in a container and freeze.		❖ Cut it up into pieces, put the butter in a bowl and whisk until you have reached the limit. ❖ Put all the butter in the container and leave it in the cooler for at least four hours. ❖ Serve and enjoyy your Strawberry Sorbet!

97) BLUEBERRY MUFFINS

Preparation Time: 1 hour	Cooking Time:	Servings: 3
✓ 1/2 cup of Blueberries ✓ 3/4 cup of Teff Flour ✓ 3/4 cup of Spelt Flour ✓ 1/3 cup of Agave Syrup		✓ 1/2 teaspoon of Pure Sea Salt ✓ 1 cup of Coconut Milk ✓ 1/4 cup Sea Moss Gel seed oil (optional, check information)
❖ Preheat our oven to 365 degrees Fahrenheit. ❖ Grate or line up 6 standard muffin cups. ❖ Add the yeast, sifter flour, sifter mashed potato, nut milk, peanut butter and agave juice to a large bowl.		❖ Put them in order for a while. ❖ Add the blueberries to the mixture and mix well. ❖ Divide muffin batter among 6 muffin cups. ❖ Bake for 30 minutes until golden brown. ❖ Serve and enjoy your Blueberry Muffins!

98) BANANA STRAWBERRY ICE CREM

Preparation Time:	Cooking Time: 4 Hours	Servings: 5
✓ 1 cup of Strawberry*. ✓ 5 quartered Baby Bananas*. ✓ 1/2 Avocado, chopped		✓ 1 tablespoon of Agave syrup ✓ 1/4 cup of Homemade Walnut Milk
❖ Put all the ingredients in and let them dry well. ❖ Taste. If so, add more milk or agave syrup if you want it to be more full-bodied.		❖ Place in a container with a lid and let crush for at least 5-6 hours. ❖ Serve it up and enjoy your creamy Bana Strawberry Ice!

Useful Tips: If you don't fresh berries or banas, you can use frozen ones. You can use as much fruit as you want, but make sure you use only fresh fruit. The fat in Avocado helps make a creamier consissitency. If you don't have homemade nut milk, you can substitute it with homemade sheep's milk.

99) CHOCOLATE CREAM HOMEMADE WHIPPED

Preparation Time: 10 Minutes.	Cooking Time:	Servings: 1 Cup
✓ 1 cup of Aquafaba		✓ 1/4 cup of Agave Syrup
❖ Add Agave Syrup and Aquafaba into a bowl. ❖ Mix to the height speed about 5 minutes with a mixer stand o 10 to 15 minutes with a mixer hand.		❖ Serve and enjoy our Homemade Whipped Cream!

Useful Tips: Remain in the refrigerator if not using immediately. The whipped cream will become Aquafaba consistency eventually, until set.

100)   "CHOCOLATE" PUDDING.

	Cooking Time: 20 Minutes.	Servings: 4

✓ 1 to 2 cups of Black Sapote ✓ 1/4 cup agave syrup ✓ 1/2 cup of soaked Brazil Nuts (overnight or at least 3 hours)	✓ 1 tbsp of Hemp Seeds ✓ 1/2 cup of Spring Water

	❖ Place all ingredients in a blender and blend until smooth. ❖ Serve and enjoy our chocolate pudding!
Directions: ❖ Cut 1 to 2 cups of Black Sapote in half. ❖ Remove all the seeds. You should have 1 cup ou full of fruit de-seeded.	

101)   WALNUT MUFFINS

Preparation Time:	Cooking Time: 1 hour	Servings: 6

✓ Dry ingredients: ✓ 1 1/2 cups of Spell or Teff Flour ✓ 1/2 teaspoon of Pure Sea Salt ✓ 3/4 cup of Date Syrup ✓ What's the big deal? ✓ 2 medium pureed Burro Banas	✓ ¼ cup of ground soybean oil ✓ ¾ cup of Homemade Walnut Milk * ✓ 1 tablespoon of Key Lime Juice ✓ Ingredients for filling: ✓ ½ cup of chopped Walnuts (plus extra for decorating) ✓ 1 banana burrita

	❖ Add the filling ingredients and fry. ❖ Place our beater in the 12 muffin cups and fill them with a knob of butter. ❖ Bake 22 to 26 mnutes until brown. ❖ Allow to cool for 10 minutes. ❖ Serve and enjoy your Bana Nut Muffins!
Directions: ❖ Preheat the oven to 400 degrees. ❖ Take a muffin tray and grease 12 cups or line with cupcake liners. ❖ Place all dry ingredients in a large bowl and mix well. ❖ Add all the ingredients to a larger bowl and mix it with the Bin Laden. 5. Mix the ingredients from the two bowls into one container. Be careful not to over mix.	

102)   WALNUT CHEESECAKE MANGO

	Cooking Time: 4 hours 30 minutes	Servings: 8

Ingredients: ✓ 2 cups of Brazil Nuts ✓ 5 to 6 Dates ✓ 1 tablespoon of Sea Moss Gel (check information) ✓ 1/4 cup of agave syrup ✓ 1/4 teaspoon salt Pure Sea ✓ 2 tablespoons of Lime Juice ✓ 1 1/2 cups of Homemade Walnut Milk *	**Ingredients:** Crust: ✓ 1 1/2 cups of quartered Dates 1/4 cup of Agave Syrup ✓ 1 1/2 cups of Coconut Flakes ✓ 1/4 teaspoon of Pure Sea Salt ✓ Toppings: ✓ Mango of Sliced ✓ Sliced strawberries

	❖ Place the filling on top of the butter, wrap it with aluminum foil or a food container and let it rest for 3 to 4 hours in the refrigerator. ❖ Take out from the baking form and garnish with toppings. ❖ Serve and enjoy our Mango Nut Cheesecake!
Directions: ❖ Place all crust ingredients in a processor and blend for 30 seconds. ❖ Prepare a baking sheet with a sheet of parchment and roll out the loose dough with butter. ❖ Place the Mango sliced across the crust and freeze for 10 minutes. ❖ Place all glass pieces in a bowl until done.	

Useful Tips: If you don't have homemade nut milk, you can use Homemade hemp seed milk.

103) BLACKBERRY JAM

Cooking Time: 4 hours and 30 minutes	**Servings: 1 cup**

✓ 3/4 cup of Blackberries ✓ 1 tablespoon lime juice Key	✓ 3 tablespoons of Agave Syrup ✓ ¼ cup of Sea Moss Gel + extra 2 tablespoons (check information)
❖ Place blackberries in a medium saucepan and cook over low heat. ❖ Stir the blackberries until the liquid is gone. ❖ Once the berries are picked, use your blender to chop up the larger pieces. If you don't have a blender, put the mixture in an immersion blender, mix it well, and then put it back in the oven.	❖ Add Sea Moss Gel, Key Lime Juice and Agave Syrup to the mixture. Simmer and stir well until dry. ❖ Remove from heat and let sit for 10 minutes. ❖ Serve with pieces or flat bread. ❖ Enjoy your jam!

Useful Tips: If you don't have Sea Moss Gel, you can omit it. However, the gel gives your skin a thinner, more durable look. Blackberries have a natural pectin, which can have a similar effect. Store this Blackberry Jam in a glass jar with a lid in the refrigerator for 2 to 3 weeks. Do not store in extreme temperatures!

104) BLACKBERRY BARS

Cooking Time: 1 Hour 20 Minutes	**Servings: 4**

✓ 3 Burro Banas or 4 Baby Banas ✓ 1 cup of Spelt Flour ✓ 2 cups of Quinoa Flakes ✓ 1/4 cup of Agave Syrup	✓ 1/4 teaspoon of Pure Sea Salt ✓ 1/2 cup of Grape Seed Oil ✓ 1 cup of prepared Blackberry Jam
❖ Set your oven to 350 degrees Fahrenheit. ❖ Mash the bananas with a fork in a large bowl. ❖ Combine Agave Syrup and Grape Seed Oil with the puree and mix well. ❖ Add the Spelt flour and Quinoa flakes. Knead the dough until it becomes sticky to your finger. ❖ Prepare a 9x9-inch basket with a parchment lid. ❖ Take 2/3 of the dough and roll it out with your fingers over the parchment pan pan.	❖ Spread Blackberry Jam over the dough. ❖ Crumble the rice and place it on the plate. ❖ Bake for 20 minutes. ❖ Remove from oven and let cool for 10-15 minutes. ❖ Cut into small pieces. ❖ Experience and enjoy our Blackberry Bars!

Useful Tips: You can keep this Blackberry Bar in the refrigerator for 5-6 days or in the freezer for up to 3 months.

105) SqUASH PIE.

Cooking Time: 2 hours 30 Minutes	**Servings: 6-8**

✓ 2 Butternut Squashes ✓ 1 1/4 cups of spelt flour ✓ 1/4 cup of dry sugar ✓ 1/4 cup of Agave Syrup ✓ 1 teaspoon of Allspice.	✓ 1 teaspoon of Pure Sea Salt ✓ 1/4 cup soy water ✓ 1/3 cup of fat seed oil ✓ 1/4 cup hemp seed milk Homemade *
❖ Rinse and peel butternut pumpkins. ❖ Cut them in half and use a spoon to de-sed. ❖ Cut the meat into one piece and place in a glass container. ❖ Cover the squash in Spring Water and boil it for 20-25 minutes until coooked. ❖ Turn off the oven and mash the cooked squash. ❖ Add the date sugar, agave syrup, 1/8 pure sea salt, and homemade milk and mix everything together. ❖ Crust: ❖ Preheat your oven to 350 degrees Fahrenheit. ❖ In a bowl, add spelt flour, 1/2 teaspoon of Pure Sea Salt, Spring Water, and Grape Sed Oil and mix.	❖ Reduce the rice into a loaf. Add more water or flour if needed. Let stand for 5 minutes. ❖ Spread out Spelt Flour on a piece of parchment paper. ❖ Roll out on rolling pin, adding more flour to prevent sticking. ❖ Place the dough in a cake pan and bake in the oven for 10 minutes. ❖ Remove the butter from the oven, add the filling and bake for another 40 minutes. ❖ Remove the cake and let it rest for 30 minutes until cool. ❖ Serve enjoy your Squash Pie!

106) WALNUT MILK HOMEMADE

	Cooking Time: minimum 8 hours	Servings: 4 cups
✓ 1 cup fresh walnuts ✓ 1/8 teaspoon of Pure Sea Salt	✓ 3 cups of spring water + extra for soaking	

Directions: ❖ Place new Walnuts in a bag and fill it with three tablespoons of water. ❖ Take the Walnuts for an hour and a half. ❖ Drain and rinse nuts with warm water.	❖ Add the soaked walnuts, puree and three times the spring water to a blender. ❖ Mix well till smooth. ❖ Stretch it out if you need to. ❖ Enjoy your homemade nut milk!

107) AqUAFABA

	Cooking Time: 2 Hours 30 minutes	Servings: 2-4 cups
✓ 1 bag of Garbanzo beans ✓ 1 teaspoon of Pure Sea Salt	✓ 6 cups of Spring Water + extra for soaking	

Directions: ❖ Place the chickpeas in a large pot, add the soy water and pure sea salt. Bring to a boil. ❖ Remove from heat and allow to soak 30 to 40 minutes. ❖ Strain the Garbanzo Beans and add 6 cups of water. ❖ Boil for 1 hour and 30 minutes on medium heat.	❖ Filter the Garbanzo beans. This filtered water is Aquafaba. ❖ Pour Aquafaba into a glass jar with a lid and place in the refrigerator. ❖ After cooling, the Aquafaba becomes thicker. If it is too thick, boil for 10-20 mnutes.

Useful Tips: Aquafaba is a good alternative for an egg: 2 tablespoons of Aquafaba = 1 egg white; 3 tablespoons of Aquafaba = 1 egg.

108) MILK HOMEMADE HEMPSEED

	Cooking Time: 2 hours	Servings: 2 cups
✓ 2 tablespoons of Hemp Seeds ✓ 2 tablespoons of Agave Syrup	✓ 1/8 teaspoon pure salt ✓ 2 cups of Spring Water Fruits (optional)*.	

❖ Place all ingredients, except the fruit, in the blender. ❖ Blend them for two minutes. ❖ Add fruits and resin for 30 to 50 minutes.	❖ Store milk in a refrigerator until old. ❖ Enjoy your Homemade Hempsed Milk!

109) OIL SPICY INFUSION

	Cooking Time: 24 Hours	Servings: 1 cup
✓ 1 tablespoon of crushed Cayenne Pepper	✓ 3/4 cup of Grape Seed Oil	

Directions: ❖ Fill a glass with a lid or bottle with grape oil. ❖ Add crushed Cayenne Pepper to the jar/bottle.	❖ Close and allow food to cool for at least 24 hours. ❖ Add it to a dinner party and enjoy our Spicy Infuse oil!

110)   ITALIAN INFUSED OIL

	Cooking Time: 24 hours	**Servings:** 1 cup
✓ 1 teaspoon of Oregano. ✓ 1 teaspoon of Basil	✓ 1 pinch of salt Pure Sea ✓ 3/4 cup of Grape seed oil	
❖ Fill a glass jar with a lid or container with grape oil. ❖ Mix the seasonings and add them to the rice and lettuce.	❖ Shake and let the oil steep for at least 24 hours. ❖ Add it to a dish and enjoy your Italian Infused Oil!	

111)   GARLIC INFUSED OIL

	Cooking Time: 24 hours	**Servings:** 1 cup
✓ 1/2 teaspoon of Dill ✓ 1/2 teaspoon of Ginger Powder ✓ 1 tablespoon of Onion Powder.	✓ 1/2 teaspoon of Pure Sea Salt ✓ 3/4 cup of fat seed oil	
❖ Fill a glass jar or squeeze bottle with grapeseed oil. ❖ Add the seasonings to the jar/bottle.	❖ Shake and let oil infuse for at least 24 hours. ❖ Add it to a dish and add your "Garlic". Infused Oil!	

112)   PAPAYA SEEDS MANGO DRESSING

	Cooking Time: 10 minutes	**Servings:** 1/2 Cup
✓ 1 cup of chopped Mango ✓ 1 tsp of Ground Papaya Seeds ✓ 1 teaspoon of Basil ✓ 1 teaspoon of Onion Powder	✓ 1 teaspoon of Agave Syrup ✓ 2 tablespoons of lemon juice ✓ 1/4 cup of grape oil ✓ 1/4 teaspoon salt Pure Sea	
❖ Prepare and place all ingredients into the mixture. ❖ Blend for one minute until smoth.	❖ Add it to a plate and enjoy our Papaya Seed Mango Dress5ng!	

113)   BLUEBERRY SMOOTHIE

Preparation Time: 10 minutes		**Servings:** 2
✓ 2 cups of frozen blueberries ✓ 1 small banana	✓ 1½ cups unsweetened almond milk ✓ ¼ cup ice cubes	
❖ Place all ingredients in a high speed blender and pulse until creamy.	❖ Pour the smoothie into two glasses and serve immediately.	

114)   RASPBERRY AND TOFU SMOOTHIE

Preparation Time: 10 minutes		**Servings:** 2
✓ 1½ cups of fresh raspberries ✓ 6 ounces of firm silken tofu, pressed and drained ✓ 4-5 drops of liquid stevia	✓ 1 cup of coconut cream ✓ ¼ cup ice, crushed	
❖ Place all ingredients in a high speed blender and pulse until creamy.	❖ Pour the smoothie into two glasses and serve immediately.	

115) BEET AND STRAWBERRY SMOOTHIE

Preparation Time: 10 minutes		**Servings: 2**
✓ 2 cups frozen strawberries, pitted and chopped ✓ ⅔ cup roasted and frozen beet, chopped ✓ 1 teaspoon fresh ginger, peeled and grated		✓ 1 teaspoon fresh turmeric, peeled and grated ✓ ½ cup of fresh orange juice ✓ 1 cup unsweetened almond milk
❖ Place all ingredients in a high speed blender and pulse until creamy.		❖ Pour the smoothie into two glasses and serve immediately.

116) KIWI SMOOTHIE

Preparation Time: 10 minutes		**Servings: 2**
✓ 4 kiwis ✓ 2 small bananas, peeled ✓ 1½ cups unsweetened almond milk		✓ 1-2 drops of liquid stevia ✓ ¼ cup ice cubes
❖ Place all ingredients in a high speed blender and pulse until creamy.		❖ Pour the smoothie into two glasses and serve immediately.

117) PINEAPPLE AND CARROT SMOOTHIE

Preparation Time: 10 minutes		**Servings: 2**
✓ 1 cup frozen pineapple ✓ 1 large ripe banana, peeled and sliced ✓ ½ tablespoon fresh ginger, peeled and chopped ✓ ¼ teaspoon ground turmeric		✓ 1 cup unsweetened almond milk ✓ ½ cup fresh carrot juice ✓ 1 tablespoon fresh lemon juice
❖ Place all ingredients in a high speed blender and pulse until creamy.		❖ Pour the smoothie into two glasses and serve immediately.

118) OATMEAL AND ORANGE SMOOTHIE

Preparation Time: 10 minutes		**Servings: 4**
✓ ⅔ cup of rolled oats ✓ 2 oranges, peeled, seeded and cut into sections ✓ 2 large bananas, peeled and sliced		✓ 2 cups of unsweetened almond milk ✓ 1 cup ice cubes, crushed
❖ Place all ingredients in a high speed blender and pulse until creamy.		❖ Pour the smoothie into four glasses and serve immediately.

119) PUMPKIN SMOOTHIE

Preparation Time: 10 minutes	**Cooking Time:**	**Servings: 2**
✓ 1 cup homemade pumpkin puree ✓ 1 medium banana, peeled and sliced ✓ 1 tablespoon maple syrup ✓ 1 teaspoon ground flax seeds		✓ ½ teaspoon ground cinnamon ✓ ¼ teaspoon ground ginger ✓ 1½ cups unsweetened almond milk ✓ ¼ cup ice cubes
❖ Place all ingredients in a high speed blender and pulse until creamy.		❖ Pour the smoothie into two glasses and serve immediately.

120) RED FRUIT AND VEGETABLE SMOOTHIE

Preparation Time: 10 minutes	Cooking Time:		Servings: 2
✓ ½ cup fresh raspberries ✓ ½ cup fresh strawberries ✓ ½ red bell pepper, seeded and chopped ✓ ½ cup red cabbage, chopped		✓ 1 small tomato ✓ 1 cup of water ✓ ½ cup of ice cubes	
❖ Place all ingredients in a high speed blender and pulse until creamy.		❖ Pour the smoothie into two glasses and serve immediately.	

121) KALE SMOOTHIE

Preparation Time: 10 minutes	Cooking Time:		Servings: 2
✓ 3 stalks of fresh cabbage, cut and chopped ✓ 1-2 celery stalks, chopped ✓ ½ avocado, peeled, pitted and chopped		✓ ½ inch ginger root, chopped ✓ ½ inch turmeric root, chopped ✓ 2 cups of coconut milk	
❖ Place all ingredients in a high speed blender and pulse until creamy.		❖ Pour the smoothie into two glasses and serve immediately.	

122) GREEN TOFU SMOOTHIE

Preparation Time: 10 minutes	Cooking Time:		Servings: 2
✓ 1½ cups cucumber, peeled and coarsely chopped ✓ 3 cups fresh spinach ✓ 2 cups of frozen broccoli ✓ ½ cup silken tofu, drained and pressed		✓ 1 tablespoon fresh lime juice ✓ 4-5 drops of liquid stevia ✓ 1 cup unsweetened almond milk ✓ ½ cup ice, crushed	
❖ Place all ingredients in a high speed blender and pulse until creamy.		❖ Pour the smoothie into two glasses and serve immediately.	

123) GRAPE AND CHARD SMOOTHIE

Preparation Time: 10 minutes	Cooking Time:		Servings: 2
✓ 2 cups of green grapes without seeds ✓ 2 cups fresh beets, cut and chopped ✓ 2 tablespoons of maple syrup		✓ 1 teaspoon fresh lemon juice ✓ 1½ cups of water ✓ 4 ice cubes	
❖ Place all ingredients in a high speed blender and pulse until creamy.		❖ Pour the smoothie into two glasses and serve immediately.	

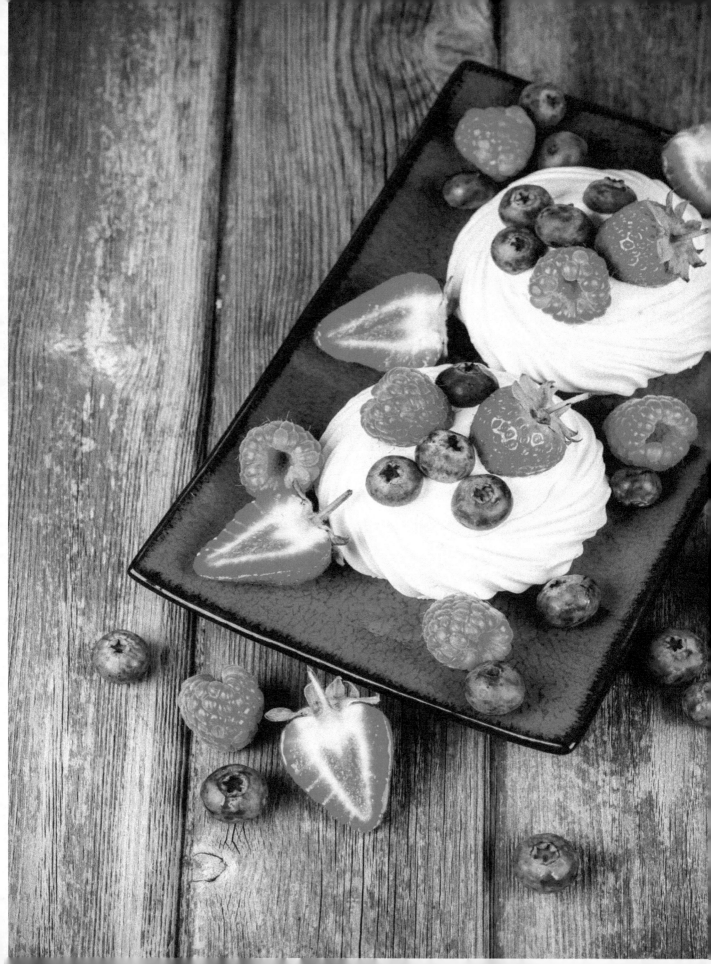

Bibliography

FROM THE SAME AUTHOR

THE ALKALINE DIET *Cookbook* - 120+ Easy-to-Follow Recipes for Beginners to start a Healthier Lifestyle!

THE ALKALINE DIET FOR BEGINNERS *Cookbook* - 120+ Super Easy Recipes to Start a Healthier Lifestyle! The Best Recipes You Need to Jump into the Alkaline and Anti-inflammatory Diet!

THE ALKALINE DIET FOR MEN *Cookbook* - The Best 120+ Recipes to Stay HEALTHY and FIT with Alkaline Diet!

THE ALKALINE DIET FOR WOMEN *Cookbook* - The Best 120+ recipes to stay TONE and HEALTHY! Reboot your Metabolism before Summer with the Lightest Alkaline Meals!

THE ALKALINE DIET FOR KIDS *Cookbook* - The Best 120+ recipes for children, tested BY Kids FOR Kids! Stay really HEALTHY with one of the most complete diet, HAVING FUN!

THE ALKALINE DIET FOR TWO *Cookbook* - 220+ Easy-to-Follow Recipes for Dad and Kids to start a Healthier Lifestyle! Stay HEALTHY and FIT making your meals together, HAVING FUN!

THE ALKALINE DIET FOR COUPLE *Cookbook* - 220+ Simple Recipes to make together! Stay HEALTHY and Eat Delicious Meals with the most complete guide about the kitchen for two!

THE ALKALINE DIET FOR MUM *Cookbook* - The Best 220+ Recipes For Mum and Kids to start a Healthier Lifestyle! HAVE FUN preparing these delicious and alkaline meals with your family!

Conclusion

Thanks for reading "The Alkaline Diet FOR MEN Cookbook"!

Follow the right habits it is essential to have a healthy Lifestyle, and the Alkaline diet is the best solution!

I hope you liked this Cookbook!

I wish you to achieve all your goals!

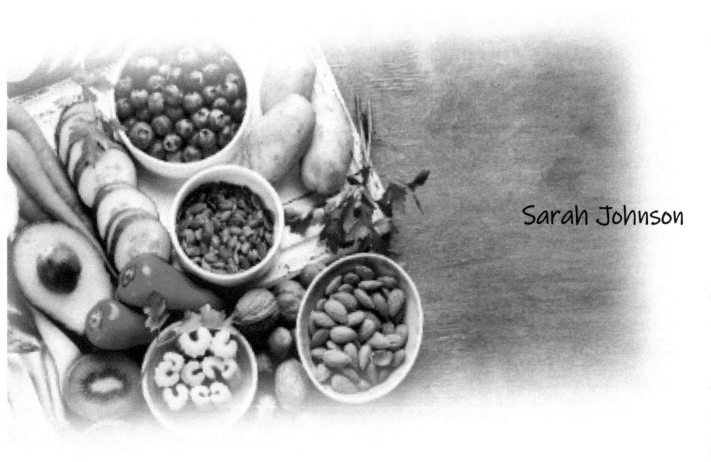

Sarah Johnson

CPSIA information can be obtained
at www.ICGtesting.com
Printed in the USA
BVHW011448120521
607126BV00005B/648